FINANCIAL MANAGEMENT
OF THE **VETERINARY** PRACTICE

FINANCIAL MANAGEMENT

OF THE **VETERINARY** PRACTICE

Justin Chamblee, CPA
Max Reiboldt, CPA

Reviewed by Nikki L. Quenette, CPA, CMA

American Animal Hospital Association Press
12575 West Bayaud Avenue
Lakewood, Colorado 80228
800-252-2242 or 303-986-2800
press.aaha.org

Library of Congress Cataloging-in-Publication Data

Chamblee, Justin.
  Financial management of the veterinary practice / Justin Chamblee, Max Reiboldt.
     p. ; cm.
  Includes bibliographical references.
  ISBN 978-1-58326-124-8 (pbk. : alk. paper)
  1. Veterinary medicine—Practice. 2. Veterinary medicine—Finance. I. Reiboldt, J. Max. II. American Animal Hospital Association. III. Title.
  [DNLM:1. Financial Management—methods. 2. Veterinary Medicine—economics. 3. Hospitals, Animal—economics. 4. Practice Management, Medical—economics. SF 756.4 C455f 2010]
  SF756.4.C43 2010
  636.089068′1--dc22
                              2010015447

Book design by Erin Johnson Design

A version of Figures 3.1, 3.2, and 3.3 first appeared in *Financial Management of the Medical Practice* (2002), published by the American Medical Association Press. Republished with permission.

Printed in the United States of America

11 12 / 10 9 8 7 6 5 4 3 2

Contents

Preface

This book on financial management is written for owners of the veterinary practice—the guardian of the animals for whom we are responsible—who often play an integral role in managing their businesses. The veterinarians we know love the animals they treat much more than they do managing their businesses. However, these two roles are inextricably intertwined, because a practice must be fiscally viable and sustainable for veterinarians to provide services. Even veterinarians who choose to be employed rather than business owners have fiscal accountability to the practices that employ them so that they can offer employment opportunities as well as veterinary care in a crowded marketplace.

The typical veterinary practice is a million-dollar operation that handles the care of numerous patients, the concerns of many clients, and the livelihood of several employees. The guidance offered in these pages is based on principles of sound financial management that apply to any small business, which is how most veterinary practices are classified. Implementing these recommendations in their business operations will give owners and managers the greatest opportunities for success in a highly competitive environment.

An important aspect of veterinary practice management is monitoring the finances of the organization. Typically, those who are responsible are generalists with broad skill sets in business operations, not accountants or financial managers. Monitoring and observing historical and current data allow the practice owner to make informed decisions.

Financial management of the veterinary practice encompasses gathering data, interpreting data, and appropriately responding. The savvy business owner will understand the nuances of data, the information yielded, and the applications that must be made to achieve a viable business organization. "Good" information does not necessarily guarantee "good" decisions, but it dramatically increases the odds that they will be made.

The purpose of this book is to help practice owners attain a sufficient level of understanding of the financial aspects of practice management to successfully function in this position. Filled with charts, checklists, examples, and sample reports, this book presents the necessary tools and fundamentals to assist the generalist owner.

The authors recognize that the veterinary practice owner may or may not have formal accounting training. The objective is to provide foundational information to nonfinancial managers that can be enhanced or supported by the accounting professionals selected to serve the practice. With a strong foundation, the generalist business owner will provide the practice with sound operational processes and fiscal stability—in addition to providing excellent veterinary care.

Acknowledgments

Books written by employees of the Coker Group are always touched by many people, both inside and outside of our organization. This work is no exception.

We express our appreciation to Nikki Quenette of Quenette Veterinary Consulting for her contributions to this book. Her expertise in the field of veterinary medicine and practice management, reflected in this book's content, will undoubtedly contribute to the success of many practices. Elise Lacher, of Strategic Veterinary Consulting, also served as a consultant for this work and provided her special perspective on financial management of veterinary practices.

We give special thanks to the contributions made by veterinarians in general practice whom we interviewed: Ray E. Habermann, DVM, Foothills Veterinary Clinic, Dawsonville, Georgia; Jim FitzSimons, DVM, Cumming Veterinary Clinic, Cumming, Georgia; and Margret Nessman, DVM, Muskego Animal Hospital, Muskego, Wisconsin. Thank you for taking time out of your busy days to work with us to enhance our understanding of the workings of veterinary practices.

In addition to the primary authors, Max Reiboldt and Justin Chamblee, Aimee Greeter, Jeffery Daigrepont, and John Reiboldt contributed their financial and technological expertise to this project.

Kay Stanley, who has contributed to the more than 50 books Coker has created since its publishing initiatives began in the early 1990s, has served as editor and project manager. Cynthia McWhorter transcribed hours of dictation with her speedy and competent hands. Based on their financial acuity, Cathy Dyer and Rick Langosch developed many spreadsheets, tables, and figures to illustrate financial concepts. Ayanna Parks is an important contributor, with her expertise in technology and skillful writing style.

Finally, we appreciate the confidence of Bess Maher, AAHA Press acquisitions editor, in supporting this project. Bess, you are the consummate professional!

CHAPTER 1

Foundational Elements of Financial Management and Reporting Standards

Sound financial management includes attention to reporting standards, which in turn requires a basic understanding of financial statements and business-accounting theories and terminology. The term reporting standards can take on many meanings, but in its basic form it refers to a foundational structure for the development and preparation of financial statements. This could mean internal consistency (within a practice), or adherence to specific accounting regulations as promulgated by entities such as the Financial Accounting Standards Board (FASB). For most veterinary practices, it is the former. This chapter first explores the key concepts for the veterinary practice in understanding financial statements. Next, it considers reporting and compilation of financial statements. It also touches on the subject of financial analysis: how to interpret financial statements. Putting it all together, it then offers a brief case study that demonstrates the value of the lessons a veterinary practice owner can learn from accurate reporting and regular analysis.

UNDERSTANDING FINANCIAL STATEMENTS

A clear understanding of the veterinary practice's financial statements requires a review of four major areas: (1) the theories, (2) the purpose, (3) the practicality, and (4) the effect of financial reporting.

Understanding the Theories

Financial management of most veterinary practices requires neither extensive accounting experience nor specialized training or an accounting degree. Most veterinary practices, whatever their size, can be managed financially without the assistance of sophisticated accounting professionals. However, larger practices may require a higher level of financial knowledge and oversight. Regardless of the size of the practice, certain financial responsibilities are typically outsourced to third-party professionals. These include primarily tax preparation and advice, valuations of practices, and other larger financial issues.

An explanation of certain basic terms will assist the average veterinary practice in meeting its financial management needs:

- **Summary of chart of accounts**. A detailed list of all accounts regularly used in the normal course of business, including balance sheets and profit and loss statements. The majority of accounts listed on the chart of accounts will be similar to those used in other industries (i.e., cash, accounts payable, revenue, salaries, rent, etc.), but there may be some accounts that are unique to the veterinary industry.

- **Profit and loss (P&L) statement.** Report detailing revenue minus expenses to show the net income during that period. Also known as an "income statement," the P&L statement is the core financial report and covers a specific period of time (usually no less than one month).

- **Balance sheet.** A statement of the financial condition of the practice listing its assets, liabilities, and owner's equity at a specific point in time. The balance sheet does not encompass any predetermined number of months or years.

- **Cash flow statement.** Report showing the sources of the practice's incoming cash and the uses of that cash. Sources of cash include such items as net income and increases in debt (wherein proceeds from the debt are contributed to the practice in the form of cash). The uses of cash include debt reduction and purchases of capital equipment and supplies. Normal overhead expenses are also uses of cash but are included in net income. (See Table 3.1 in Chapter 3 for a more detailed sample income statement for the veterinary practice.)

- **Assets.** Everything of value owned by the company or corporation. Current assets are items that will be consumed within a short period of time, often one year, while fixed or long-term assets have value extending longer than one year.

- **Liabilities.** The practice's debts; that is, money that is owed to lenders or other parties. Liabilities can include short-term debts, such as accounts payable, as well as long-term debts, such as a mortgage on the practice's facility.

- **Equity.** Assets minus liabilities. On a more theoretical basis, the term connotes the net worth of the business. Sometimes equity is also referred to as "net book value."

The owner or manager of a veterinary practice (typically not a trained accountant or financial analyst) should understand the "big picture" of these financial terms and financial statements. Once these basics are understood, financial interpretation can begin. This often requires applying common sense more than theory, because although accounting may be "black and white," there are no hard and fast rules about the operation of a veterinary practice, or of any other business.

Financial Reporting Accounting Methodologies

In financial reporting there is one decision that must be made at the outset, as the answer affects just about every report to be produced and analyzed for the practice. That question concerns the method of accounting to be used. In basic terms, there are two ways to account for the operations of the veterinary practice, cash and accrual. There are pros and cons to both methods.

Cash-based accounting calls for recognition of revenue when cash is *received* and recognition of expenses when cash is *expended* or *paid*. Small businesses (and most veterinary practices) often use a cash basis of accounting.

In most small businesses, the phrase "cash is king" is very relevant. Cash-based accounting, which reflects revenue based on actual monies received, has more immediate relevance for veterinary practices than does accrual-based accounting. It allows practice owners and managers to see the effects of day-to-day operations more clearly than is generally possible with the accrual method. The owner or manager should be careful to pay the practice's expenses on a timely basis to avoid overstating its net income. When the financial statements do not reflect true operating performance, the inevitable day of reckoning will come. If cash-based (or modified cash-based) methods are used, it is essential to present an accurate and timely depiction of both revenue received and expenses paid.

Accrual-based accounting considers revenue when it is *earned* and expenses when they are *incurred*—for example, when services are performed and goods are used. Sometimes a veterinary practice will make accrual-based entries in its accounting system. These may be items such as accounts payable and depreciation. Other practices even maintain some level of inventory and/or accounts receivable on their books. In these cases, the practice's external tax accountant will obtain the accounting records annually and adjust them to a cash basis of accounting to complete the tax return.

An important part of accrual-based accounting is depreciation. *Depreciation* is the recognition of the cost of an asset, such as equipment or buildings, whose value (i.e., useful life) is extended beyond the period being measured (usually a month or a year). To recognize the value of the asset over an extended period, it is most appropriate to *depreciate its cost*. For example, the veterinary practice purchases an automobile at a cost of $30,000. That automobile is deemed to have a *useful life* of five years. Thus, the cost of the automobile is recognized over the five-year period (its useful life), not just in the period when it was purchased.

There are numerous methods of depreciation. The simplest is the straight-line basis, wherein the cost of the asset is recognized evenly over its useful life. Thus, a $30,000 automobile depreciated over five years would recognize depreciation at the rate of $6,000 per year ($30,000 divided into 5 equal parts, or $6,000). Another method used in small businesses is the Modified Accelerated Cost Recovery System (MACRS), an accelerated depreciation method required by the U.S. income tax code. Under MACRS, the depreciation is accelerated so that more of the cost is recognized in the first several years, and less near the end, of the asset's useful life. For example, using the straight-line method, the depreciation of the automobile was $6,000 in the first year, whereas using MACRS, it could be $12,000. In smaller practices, the external tax accountant usually handles depreciation issues and is the best source of information if the owner or manager has questions about the depreciation of certain assets.

As a general rule, accrual-based accounting is considered more accurate than cash-based accounting, because it considers the financial effects not when revenue is received or expenses paid but when services are performed or goods used. The purchase of supplies provides a good example. If a veterinary practice purchases supplies in bulk and incurs a substantial cost when doing so, but uses the cash basis of accounting, the practice will appear to have performed poorly in the month when the supplies were purchased. But the supplies will be used over time, not just during that month. In the following months the financial performance will look better than it really is because the cost of the supplies being used will not show up as an expense. Accordingly, in a cash-based system there will be many peaks and valleys. Under the accrual-based method of accounting, the supplies purchased would have been put into inventory (an asset account) and the expense would have been recognized as the supplies were actually used. Thus, the use of the supplies would match when the expense was incurred. This helps to smooth out the financial performance of a practice, on paper. Over time, the revenue and expenses will be the same in both systems.

Very few veterinary practices use accrual-based accounting because of its complexity, but it is important to understand its benefits in case there are valid reasons to implement it at a particular time or for a particular practice. When choosing an appropriate method of accounting, practice owners and managers should consider both the pros and cons of each approach. Accrual-based accounting should be used for larger entities, and the Internal Revenue Service requires this method for all companies with gross revenues exceeding $10 million per year. The threshold is actually lower for most companies, but those that provide a service (such as a veterinary practice) may meet the higher threshold.

(handwritten margin notes: "services / supplies / drug)" *"Per vet (emergency vs non emergency / supplies / Drug)"*

Understanding the Purpose

The purpose of financial statements and other financial interpretive analyses is to allow the owners and managers of the practice to properly review what has happened in the period being measured. Why is this important? Quite simply, timely reporting and analysis enable owners and managers to make good decisions about practice operations. Accurate financial statements—whether cash or accrual based—assuming that business owners and managers understand them, may be the most useful tools for determining current performance, forecasting future performance, and making important management decisions. Reflective analysis of financial information through a consistent review of financial statements should be part of the monthly routine of the veterinary practice owner or manager. Key employees, including department heads and other staff members, should also be part of this review.

Depending on the level of detail required by the veterinary practice's record keeping, statements may be segmented by department, definitely for revenue, and perhaps for both revenue and expense allocations. An examination of financial statements should entail a separate review of each department. For example, the boarding component of most veterinary practices should be departmentalized as a stand-alone "profit center." It is essential for the owner and each department manager to understand the mechanics of this business component. A separate income statement, for instance, could be derived exclusively for the boarding department of the veterinary practice. Revenue would be straightforward (i.e., the charges assessed to clients who boarded their pets). Expenses would be both direct and indirect: direct costs would be those specifically related to boarding, and indirect costs would be those attributable to the boarding department, such as accounting, billing, and maintenance of the facility, including rent.

The ultimate purpose of financial statements—whether as a whole or by department—is to give key personnel the necessary information to react to information about current performance and to predict and respond to future projections. An understanding of past performance will allow practice owners and managers to use these factors as a basis for predicting future trends. Accurate reporting makes it possible to base decisions on good information, which promotes good decisions and helps managers make knowledgeable projections.

Understanding the Practicality

Many nonfinancial managers shy away from review of financial statements because they lack understanding, background, or training in this area. This is unfortunate and can create difficulties for the business owner. Many veterinary business owners prefer to limit themselves to their clinical expertise—that for which they are trained—and tend to neglect the day-to-day financial management of the business. From a practical standpoint, the application of the basic concepts discussed in this chapter will help the practice owner immensely. The financial novice will be able to distinguish between areas of monetary importance and those that are relatively insignificant.

The basic financial statement review will help practice owners and managers identify trends that indicate problems or issues needing attention. Applying a day-to-day, practical approach to financial statements is very beneficial and even necessary to running a successful practice. The practice owner should not be apprehensive about lack of extensive accounting training or knowledge. Taking a practical approach rather than a technical one, this chapter and the rest of this book provide basic information and applications sufficient for the financial management of the veterinary practice.

Understanding the Effect

Financial statements provide information about many things. The balance sheet shows the condition of the business relative to the value of its assets versus its liabilities and the overall net book value (or net worth) of the business. The income statement, if done accurately, captures the performance within a defined period of time (i.e., month, quarter, or year). It reveals how the business has performed through the basic formula of revenue minus expense equals income (R − E = I), which is all that is necessary for the nonfinancial manager or owner to understand. The cash flow statement provides insight into the position of the business relative to cash flow within that period—an important part of financial management.

Review of statements provides historical insights as well as a perspective on the future, especially if similar events are allowed to occur. Further review is warranted if the income statement reflects higher than expected costs (based upon an established budget). For example, personnel is one of the largest expenses of the veterinary practice. If that cost is much higher than expected, although nothing can be done to change that history, the manager or owner of the practice can consider the appropriate actions to take to control that expense. Thus a historical review can have a positive effect on the future.

It is insufficient to just accurately report financial performance. The next—and most important—step is using the financial statements as a management tool to make sound and thoughtful business decisions.

PROPER FINANCIAL STATEMENT STRUCTURE

Table 1.1 shows the appropriate financial statement structure for the most important of all financial statements: the income statement. This is an example of a typical veterinary

Revenue - expense = Income

TABLE 1.1
Example of an Income Statement (Modified Cash Basis)

ABC VETERINARY ASSOCIATES, P.A.
Statement of Income and Expenses for the Years Ended December 31, 20XX and 20XX
See Accountant's Compilation Report

	Year 1	Year 2
INCOME		
Veterinary Services and Sales	$ 1,053,343	$ 915,950
COST OF GOODS AND SERVICES		
Supplies—Medical and Resale	189,602	164,871
Laboratory Fees	36,867	32,058
Total Cost of Goods and Services	226,469	196,929
GROSS PROFIT	$ 826,874	$ 719,021
EXPENSES		
Administrative		
Advertising	10,533	9,160
Amortization	378	329
Bank Charges and Processing Fees	17,907	15,571
Contributions	2,100	1,500
Dues and Subscriptions	1,438	1,250
Miscellaneous	6,600	5,769
Professional Services	17,250	15,000
Supplies and Postage	15,800	13,739
Taxes and Licenses	1,053	916
Travel/Meals	1,980	2,591
Total Administrative	75,040	65,825
Compensation & Benefits		
Owner Compensation	75,000	75,000
Associate Compensation	119,425	106,553
Staff Compensation	228,575	192,350
Contract Labor	7,475	6,500
Insurance	21,067	18,319
Payroll Taxes	26,470	23,016
Continuing Education	1,725	1,500
Total Compensation & Benefits	479,737	423,238
Facility		
Depreciation	37,867	32,928
Equipment Rental	1,857	1,615
Rent	63,000	63,000
Repairs and Maintenance	15,800	12,122
Telephone	7,935	6,900
Utilities	8,427	7,328
Total Facility	134,886	123,893
Total Expenses	689,662	612,955
OTHER INCOME/EXPENSE		
Interest Expense	16,521	17,495
NET INCOME	$ 120,691	$ 88,570

net worth

Example of a Balance Sheet

ABC VETERINARY ASSOCIATES, P.A.
Balance Sheet for the Years Ended December 31, 20XX and 20XX
See Accountant's Compilation Report

	Year 1	Year 2
CURRENT ASSETS		
Cash on Hand and in Banks	$ 297,535	$ 189,622
Accounts Receivable	36,023	28,000
Inventory	52,000	67,000
Total Current Assets	**385,558**	**284,622**
FIXED ASSETS		
Building	250,000	250,000
Furniture, Fixtures, and Equipment	225,181	190,181
Land	50,000	50,000
Total Cost	**525,181**	**490,181**
Less Accumulated Depreciation	349,867	312,000
Total Fixed Assets	**175,314**	**178,181**
OTHER ASSETS		
Loan Closing Costs (Net of Amortization)	22,613	22,991
TOTAL ASSETS	**$ 583,485**	**$ 485,794**
LIABILITIES AND STOCKHOLDER'S EQUITY		
CURRENT LIABILITIES		
Accounts Payable	$ 39,000	$ 50,000
Bank One Visa Card	2,000	3,000
Sales Tax Payable	1,000	2,000
Total Current Liablities	**42,000**	**55,000**
LONG-TERM LIABILITIES		
Notes Payable—Local Bank	132,000	140,000
Lease Payable—US Bancorp	5,000	7,000
Total Long-Term Liabilities	**137,000**	**147,000**
TOTAL LIABILITIES	**179,000**	**202,000**
STOCKHOLDER'S EQUITY		
Capital Stock	1	1
Stockholder's Equity	404,484	283,793
Total Stockholder's Equity	**404,485**	**283,794**
TOTAL LIABILITIES AND STOCKHOLDER'S EQUITY	**$ 583,485**	**$ 485,794**

income statement on a modified cash basis. It shows revenue (i.e., cash basis or cash received) versus expenses, all expenses being recognized as paid, with the exception of depreciation.

Table 1.2 is an example of a balance sheet. This is the second most important financial statement for the veterinary practice. Another important document—the statement of cash flows—is shown in Table 1.3. These three statements are discussed in detail below.

The source for these statements is the chart of accounts. As illustrated in Table 1.1, a chart of accounts, in the most basic sense, is a list of all the accounts in a business's general ledger. This list includes both balance sheet and income statement accounts. The American Animal Hospital Association (AAHA) has published the *AAHA Chart of Accounts*, a standard chart of accounts for veterinary practices that expands the categories shown in Table 1.1 into even more detail. Using a chart of accounts helps the veterinary practice ensure that it has meaningfully represented the source of its transactions

TABLE 1.3

Example of a Statement of Cash Flows

ABC VETERINARY ASSOCIATES, P.A.
Statement of Cash Flows for the Years Ended December 31, 20XX and 20XX
See Accountant's Compilation Report

	Year 1	Year 2
CASH FLOW FROM OPERATING ACTIVITIES		
Net Income	$ 120,691	$ 88,570
Adjustments to Reconcile Net Income to Net Cash Provided (Used) by Operating Activities		
Depreciation and Amortization	38,245	33,257
Decrease in Accounts Receivable	(8,023)	4,044
Decrease in Inventory	15,000	(12,329)
Increase (Decrease) in Accounts Payable	(12,000)	6,178
Increase (Decrease) in Taxes Payable	(1,000)	(98)
NET CASH PROVIDED BY OPERATING ACTIVITIES	**152,913**	**119,622**
CASH FLOW TO INVESTING ACTIVITIES		
Purchase of Fixed Assets—Net	(35,000)	(20,000)
CASH FLOW FROM (TO) FINANCING ACTIVITIES		
Borrowings Net of Principal Payments	(10,000)	20,000
NET CASH (TO) FINANCING ACTIVITIES	**(10,000)**	**20,000**
NET INCREASE (DECREASE) IN CASH	**107,913**	**119,622**
CASH AT BEGINNING OF YEAR	**189,622**	**70,000**
CASH AT END OF YEAR	**$ 297,535**	**$ 189,622**

and described them consistently in the financial statements. It also provides data that serve as a comparable source for benchmarking a practice's performance against that of other practices (as discussed in Chapter 5).

The Income Statement
Table 1.1, an example of an income statement, is a very basic presentation. Income from veterinary services and sales, less the cost of goods and services, results in gross profit. When the additional operating expenses are subtracted from gross profit, the result is net income.

The income statement has predictable line items. It is also noteworthy that the individual line items are compared by presenting both the prior year and current year under review. The line items are areas of expenses for typical components of operations, such as advertising, contract labor, equipment rental, insurance, interest, professional services, repairs and maintenance, and customarily the largest single expenditure, compensation. The other major expense is supplies—both medical and those for resale—which are classified as a cost of goods and services.

Stating expenses as a percentage of revenue is an extremely valuable tool to ensure proper interpretation and comparative performance. This also helps with the budgeting process. Although the statement in Table 1.1 does not indicate the corresponding percentages of expenses to revenue, these points are presented and explained later in this book.

The final net income total can also be expressed as a percentage of revenue, which is often very revealing. Comparing revenue and expenses from one year to the next shows the operational performance in detail and provides valuable information.

The Balance Sheet
The balance sheet in Table 1.2 offers a snapshot of the condition of the organization on two specific dates one year apart. Assets equal the combination of liabilities and equity, which is the basic accounting equation. This same equation can be stated in a variety of ways, just as most other mathematical problems can. For example, assets minus liabilities equals equity, and assets minus equity would equal liabilities. The data for each component (i.e., assets, liabilities, and equity) is available, and it is a matter of simply putting them together to formulate the balance sheet.[1] Like the income statement, the balance sheet shows the value of assets and amount of debt as well as shareholders' equity compared with those of the same period in the prior year. By listing the financial data for two points in time, one can see how the practice finances are improving or regressing.

Usually the balance sheet is strictly representative of the cost or basis of the assets to the owner. Thus an increase in the market value of an asset, such as real estate, is generally not represented. If it is, the increase must be based on a significant amount of substantiated evidence and documentation.

The Statement of Cash Flows

The statement of cash flows (Table 1.3) illustrates the cash that has been generated or has come into the business minus the cash that has flowed out of the business, rendering the cash total at the end of the year.

This statement shows sources and uses of cash to generate the balance at year-end. From a management perspective, the cash flow statement provides valuable insight into the use of such monies. However, many small businesses rarely use a statement of cash flows. This is both because they are slightly more complicated to derive and because, in a cash-based business, the cash flow statement presents information that is not much different from the income statement. Still, the statement of cash flows can provide valuable insights into exactly where cash is coming from and going to on a month-to-month basis.

CHARACTERISTICS OF GOOD FINANCIAL REPORTING

To provide adequate information for making good management decisions, the reporting process must be well designed and consistent. Good financial reports have the following characteristics:

- **Timeliness.** Financial statements should reflect recent historical results and be turned around quickly at the conclusion of the reporting period.
- **Accuracy.** Reliable and accurate data are essential if financial statements are to be useful for decision making. Accuracy can be ensured through an independent audit, which reviews and sanctions the statements based on generally accepted accounting principles, but most small businesses will not go to the expense of procuring an independent audit—nor should they. Often the veterinary practice will complete such a review via an accountant's compilation. This is not an independent opinion, but it does provide the assurance that the financial statements have been presented in accordance with prescribed standards. Figure 1.1 is an example of the accountant's compilation report.
- **Simplicity.** This chapter has introduced basic financial concepts, not intricate accounting detail. Although proper accounting should govern any financial statement presentation, as far as the overall reporting process is concerned, for the typical veterinary practice the reports should provide information that is easy to interpret.

- **Sufficient detail.** Although good financial reporting maintains simplicity, it should still include enough detail to enhance accuracy and decision making. The financial statements provided in the tables in this chapter do just that; they are neither too complex nor too simple. They present the financial performance and condition of the veterinary practice in a way that even the nonaccountant veterinary owner can readily understand with a limited amount of coaching and training. If more detail is needed, it can be derived from backup information and source

FIGURE 1.1

Example of the Accountant's Compilation Report

Board of Directors
ABC Veterinary Associates, P.A.
Anywhere, USA

I have compiled the accompanying balance sheet of ABC Veterinary Associates, P.A. as of December 31, 20XX and 20XX, and the related statement of income and cash flows for the years then ended, in accordance with Statements on Standards for Accounting and Review Services issued by the American Institute of Certified Public Accountants.

A compilation is limited to presenting in the form of financial statements information that is the representation of management. I have not audited or reviewed the accompanying financial statements and, accordingly, do not express an opinion or any other form of assurance on them.

Management has elected to omit substantially all of the disclosures required by generally accepted accounting principles. If the omitted disclosures were included in the financial statements, they might influence the user's conclusions about the Company's financial position, results of operations, and cash flows. Accordingly, these financial statements are not designed for those who are not informed about such matters.

January 1, 20XX

data, which encompass such things as the general ledger and subsidiary ledger reports, including an accounts receivable subledger, a fixed asset subledger, and other related reports.

- **Analytical relevance.** The information provided should be worthy of analysis, usually from a comparative standpoint. The comparisons may be with the prior year, as illustrated in the tables in this chapter, or they may be set against industry benchmarks and budgets. Industry benchmarking data and practice budgets can be important tools in analyzing financial data and are described throughout this book.

Basic financial statements should be completed on a regular basis, preferably monthly, but at least quarterly. When a standard reporting cycle is used, owners and managers will benefit by seeing operational results in a timely manner. In fact, they should review the financial performance for the prior month within five to ten business days of the end of the month. An independent accountant's compilation need not be completed monthly and may be done either quarterly or yearly.

Financial statements can help the practice owner and/or manager assess trends concisely, providing objective pictures of performance for the review period.

FINANCIAL ANALYSIS SIMPLIFIED

In recent years the level of complexity has increased in many businesses. The veterinary practice is no exception. The need for highly proficient and competent business specialists, such as CPAs and managers with MBAs, has mounted in virtually all industries. Although practice owners are enhancing their skills in financial analysis, they may lack financial training and time to devote to financial management. This calls for a simplified financial analysis process.

Financial analysis entails the ability to interpret and evaluate the relationships between various statements and, within them, specific numerical indicators. With this interpretation should come implementation of action-oriented initiatives. When a financial statement is reviewed and then analyzed, conclusions should be drawn that will affect the ongoing decision making of the organization. This concept is presented in a brief case study at the end of this chapter.

The typical financial reporting package for a practice includes the three main financial statements discussed above: the balance sheet, the income statement, and the statement of cash flows. In fact, because many veterinary practices are very small, often only the balance sheet and income statement are used. Additional reporting may be used to interpret the data in the typical financial reporting package and to draw out key areas of focus.

Financial Analysis Perspectives

Veterinary practice owners or managers who wish to use financial analysis to make good decisions will need to consider the following key principles:

- **Safeguarding assets.** A system should be in place to make sure that assets are protected and appropriately accounted for from one period to the next.
- **Pricing/fee structure.** The quantity of one good or service (usually cash) given in return for a unit of another good or service is at the core of the organization's ability to generate acceptable amounts of revenue.
- **Cost evaluation.** The process of calculating the cost of activities, products, or sales must also be considered.
- **Procurement of capital (through financing and/or investors).** Obtaining resources from the owners, providing them with a return on their investment, obtaining resources from creditors, and repaying amounts borrowed are integral to financial statement analysis. In many instances, the veterinarian is not only the owner of, but also the lender to, the practice.
- **Incremental performance.** For the veterinary practice, performance-measurement issues can be broken down by the various departments and/or profit centers. Descriptions of changes in cost, expense, investment, cash flow, revenue profit, and other related metrics are key to these evaluations.
- **Accountability via departmentalization.** Akin to incremental performance measurement is consideration of various units in the practice as departments or subsets of the entire organization. Examples are boarding, grooming, and retail sales. These profit centers may each have their own individual statement of performance, which in a small business such as a veterinary practice typically consists of just an income statement. Tracking financial performance at this level may provide additional insights into the profitability of the various service lines and allows the practice owners to make more informed decisions about which areas need improvement or expansion. Most often, departmental reporting occurs only in larger practices with an accounting department, but some basic departmental reporting can be completed in even the smallest of practices using software such as QuickBooks™.
- **Profitability analysis.** Analysis of profitability considers net income within the entire organization and/or department and may include some of the types of analysis discussed previously, including comparison with prior periods, budgeting, and industry benchmarks. When analyzing practice profitability, it is important to understand how profitability is defined in each instance. For example, profitability for a tax return can have a very different meaning from the true profitability of a practice. When examining the true profitability of a practice, certain adjustments

should be considered, including depreciation of assets (if they are being depreciated faster than their actual wear), compensation of the practice owner (if a "market" level of compensation is not being charged to the practice), any discretionary expenses paid by the practice for the owners that in most cases would not be considered true business expenses, and rent (if the owner of the practice also owns the real estate and charges a rental that is above or below market rates). These factors, and others, can affect the profitability of the practice and should be adjusted for if true profitability is being considered.

- **Return on capital analysis.** This type of analysis considers income before distributions to the suppliers of capital for a specific period in the form of a rate. As a rate, this amount is derived by dividing income by average total assets to obtain a return on capital percentage. Usually this is a percentage of earnings before interest, taxes, depreciation, and amortization (EBITDA).

Financial Analysis Procedures

Different veterinary practices may follow slightly different financial analysis procedures depending on the "key performance indicators" (KPIs) their owners and managers decide to track. Financial analysis procedures can be defined as *the steps that an individual or organization performs to analyze financial data.* KPIs are basic statistics about practice operations used to measure performance within the organization. It is a general term that relates to the key pieces of data that each individual practice chooses to focus on. KPIs may also be used to expand upon information in the financial statements, to explain changes from one period to another, and to compare one veterinary practice operation with others. Many KPIs provide important details about revenue generated by the practice—for example, an increase in revenue may be due to an increase in number of clients seen or to an increase in the average amount each client spends. Other KPIs may measure client activity, collectibility of accounts receivable, and veterinarian performance.

KPI information is readily available for most veterinary practice management systems and usually is summarized through a spreadsheet program for interpretation. Each month should be compared with other months and with the same month in the prior year in order to reveal any trends.

The sidebar "Common KPIs for the Veterinary Practice" summarizes KPIs that should be used. Other KPIs may be developed as applicable to the individual veterinary practice. For example, an entity that wants to increase the number of dental reviews completed will track this statistic each month. This would be measured for the entire practice as well as by individual veterinarian.

Common KPIs for the Veterinary Practice

- Total practice revenue by month
- Total practice transactions by month
- Average transaction charge for the practice by month
- New clients by month
- Lost clients per month
- Revenue, transactions, and average transaction charge per individual doctor per month
- Revenue by category (immunization, laboratory, etc.)
- Accounts receivable by aging classification (i.e., current, 0–30 days, 31–60 days, etc.)

In addition to the KPIs, three key areas of financial analysis should be considered (financial analysis is discussed in greater detail in Chapters 4 and 5):

- **Percentage statement analysis.** As discussed previously, the income statement should be presented as a ratio of expenses to total revenue (i.e., revenue = 100 percent). Thus, all expense categories, including major expenses incurred by the practice, will be stated as a percentage of revenue. This percentage should be compared with those of prior periods, industry benchmarks, budgeted performance, and other viable metrics. Often percentages can be another very useful indicator of financial performance along with absolute dollars. Table 3.1 provides an example of percentage statement analysis within an income statement. Percentage statement analysis is also called *common sizing* or *right sizing*.

- **Ratios.** These represent the determination of financial statement entry relationships (i.e., income statement item to income statement item, income statement item to balance sheet item, balance sheet item to balance sheet item, etc.). The fractional structure that results provides a concise reference to performance. Ratios are generally used to assess aspects of profitability, solvency, and liquidity. They are relationships of one number to another between various statements or other performance-based data, such as number of visits, and provide insight about financial performance. Ratios are explored in greater detail in Chapter 5, as they provide a concise summary of practice performance.

- **Variance analysis.** This is a method of reviewing financial statements in relation to either prior periods or budgeted amounts to determine where variances in the financial accounts are occurring and why. This analysis explicitly outlines variances between line items and brings them to the forefront. For example, if salary expense has increased significantly over what was budgeted, this warrants further investigation and documentation. From that information, management can decide how to address the problem, if it can be corrected. Thus, variance analysis may be a vital tool for the veterinary practice owner.

CASE STUDY: FINANCIAL STATEMENT ANALYSIS

Dr. John Jones owns a veterinary practice in the southeastern United States. It has operated under a basic financial analysis for some time. In a review of the financial statements of the practice for year 20XX ending in December, it became apparent that overhead had increased significantly over the prior year. This was evident by the income statement's presentation of each expense as an absolute dollar amount, accompanied by a corresponding percentage showing the relationship of each expense to revenue.

In completing the year-end financial analysis and assessing overhead, Dr. Jones realized that the nonveterinarian salary expense (i.e., cost of all support personnel in his practice) had risen significantly. The absolute dollar amount budgeted for the year for this cost was $120,000. Although the dollar amount was helpful, it was not as revealing as the cost indicated on a percentage basis of expenses. This cost, which actually ended up at $150,000 per year, was in and of itself obviously a higher amount than the amount budgeted. The amount budgeted would have been 20 percent of revenue, but the amount spent was actually closer to 25 percent of revenue—a clear excess. Thus, from the financial statements, and specifically the income statement, it became obvious that too much was being spent in this area.

Once this problem was identified, it was discovered that one reason for the excessive salary expense was the use of more part-time staff than originally planned, due to leeway given to departmental managers in making certain employment decisions. Another reason was that overtime pay was being allowed for full-time hourly nonexempt employees, and the cost had spiraled out of control. The argument could be made that if Dr. Jones had been reviewing his financials on a regular basis rather than just at year-end, he would have become aware of this problem sooner.

Although year 20XX is past and Dr. Jones cannot undo what was done, he learned a valuable lesson for the future: He now knows to complete a review of his financial statements monthly on a line-by-line basis, using both absolute dollars and percentage of revenue to spot trends. He also knows he must compare the budget with actual performance.

SUMMARY

Understanding financial statements, other related reports, and the subsequent reporting process is fundamental to the successful financial management of the veterinary practice. As basic standards are established, maintained, and adhered to, the ability to conduct sound, thorough, and accurate financial performance evaluation will increase. This can be done by the nonaccountant owner or manager of the practice (often in collaboration with the accountant/CPA professional at certain junctures). Financial statements should be reviewed with an understanding of what each account means and the kind of transactions that apply to that account. Doing so will enable the owner and manager of the practice to be much more adept at evaluating the organization's financial performance.

Note

1. Further discussion relative to this concept and how and why the basic accounting equation works would require a detailed study of the foundations of accounting, which is outside the scope of this text. There are many useful resources that provide information regarding the foundations of accounting, which is universal across all industries.

CHAPTER 2

The Revenue Cycle

The only way for an organization to remain solvent is by generating income. Any business can acquire raw materials, create finished goods, and market a product, but a successful business does all that *and* sells the good (or service) to produce income. Although a company could borrow funds from a number of sources, if it is unable to pay off its debts through the revenue it produces, the business will not be sustainable. A veterinary practice is no different from any other business entity: Income is requisite for its continued existence. Even with a steady stream of clients, a solid staff, and a central location, a veterinary practice's success is determined by the revenue it generates. This chapter analyzes the operational and financial mechanisms by which revenue is generated and the processes used to maximize revenue production.

COMPONENTS OF THE REVENUE CYCLE

Though the revenue cycle can differ from one industry or line of business to the next, certain foundational elements are present in every organization. This section analyzes these key components and relates them specifically to a veterinary practice.

Appointment Scheduling

The revenue cycle begins long before the exchange of money. To generate revenue, a business must first have people willing to purchase the goods or services it provides. In a veterinary practice, clients generally make appointments to purchase the goods and services offered. Some practices are utilizing advanced technology, such as Internet-based appointment scheduling, but the majority of practices and their clients still schedule appointments by telephone. When a client calls the practice, the appointment may be scheduled by any one of various individuals or departments, depending on the size of the practice. Some practices have designated reception or front-office staff responsible for scheduling. Smaller practices may cross-train staff members to handle appointment scheduling as well as other duties (including clinical duties). In other practices, departments rotate responsibilities, requiring most staff members to be proficient in the scheduling function.

Regardless of who is responsible for scheduling appointments, this task requires planning and foresight to effectively maximize revenue. Knowing that it generates revenue primarily from these appointments, a veterinary practice will want to make as many appointments as possible while balancing quality of care and client satisfaction. Appointments should be scheduled to allow for the greatest number of patients to be seen while allocating a reasonable amount of time to each. Scheduling to meet this goal can involve patients being dropped off, double-booking, making allowances for no-shows, and creating space for unscheduled or emergency cases. A practice should also consider how to arrange a schedule to best meet the needs of the target market. For example, practices may elect to have early morning hours or evening hours to accommodate the schedules of working professionals. This scheduling arrangement may require that the veterinarians in the practice stagger their work hours to cover all available appointment times effectively.

Because appointments are the initial step in the generation of revenue, the importance of effective scheduling cannot be overstated. To reduce the number of no-shows, practices may institute a system of telephone calls or e-mails to remind clients of their scheduled appointments. Many practices send their clients postcards or letters to remind them of upcoming dates for annual examinations, tests, immunizations, and vaccinations. These courtesy reminders help clients with the ongoing maintenance of their pets' health, but they are also a marketing tool and mechanism by which additional appointments (and subsequent revenue) are generated.

Check-In

Depending on the practice, check-in may occur in part at the time an appointment is scheduled or be done completely when a client arrives at the practice. Checking in includes updating or confirming client demographic information, such as phone number and address; completing a brief history for the new patient; and explaining the reason for the visit. Some veterinary offices are going paperless (or nearly paperless), maintaining all demographic information and records of patient visits in practice management system (PMS) software. Some practices may copy documentation and maintain paper files of information brought in when the client transfers from another practice. For the many practices that are not automated, clients may be asked at check-in to complete the postcard or letter that the practice will mail to remind them of their next regularly scheduled appointment. Automated practices may notify veterinarians electronically of the client and patient's arrival, or staff may announce the patient. In the nonautomated practice, the check-in process would include having a staff member pull the patient's medical record and notify the veterinary technician or veterinarian that the client is waiting. At this time, the patient is transferred to the care of the veterinarian, who will be responsible for the majority of the appointment.

Check-in is a time to greet the client and the patient enthusiastically. Scheduled appointments should be handled promptly, and walk-ins should receive an accurate estimate of wait time, including an offer for the client to leave the patient and return later for pickup. It is important to use check-in time to explain the practice's payment policy or changes in other procedures since the client's last visit. These types of interactions are often instrumental in achieving high client satisfaction. Clients who are highly satisfied will be more willing to return to the practice for further care for their animals. The check-in process and all client interactions should be professional and positive.

Client Compliance

After the client has checked in, the veterinarian examines the patient and determines an appropriate course of treatment. In many practices, at this point the veterinarian explains to the client what tests should be performed, what products should be used, and other procedures to be completed. The charges for each of these recommendations are also outlined at this time. The client then accepts or declines the services. By having a client agree to treatment and acknowledge the cost up front, the practice has a greater opportunity to collect for the services to be performed, as the client must prepare to pay before the procedures occur. See the section "Revenue Enhancement" for information on increasing compliance.

Charge Capture

When a patient is seen in a veterinary practice, the diagnosis and treatment (including any injections, vaccines, and pharmaceuticals given) must be recorded and the associated charges documented. This typically occurs through the use of a "travel sheet" or a "super bill." Essentially, the travel sheet lists all of the procedures/services available at the practice; as services are provided, the veterinarian marks them on the sheet. This can be either a laminated piece of paper that is reused by simply marking on it using a dry-erase marker, or a disposable piece of paper for onetime use. In most cases, it is the veterinarian's responsibility to approve and document the services to be charged.

Then the travel sheet is handed off to the front-desk staff, typically to be entered and paid for at the time services are rendered. In automated practices, this process is completed electronically using the PMS. Charge capture then entails the transfer of all proper documentation into the practice's billing system so compensation for services performed can be collected from the client. To maximize revenue, it is important that the practice capture, bill, and collect all applicable charges. Without efficient charge capture, the practice will lose revenue for services already performed, to the detriment of its bottom line.

Patient and Insurance Billing

Once all charges have been input into the billing system, the practice can collect payment from the client, which typically should occur at the time services are rendered. Clearly, this may be the most important step in the revenue cycle. Veterinary practice clients are almost always assessed their fees at the point of service, as opposed to receiving a bill at a later date. Upon completion of the patient's clinical treatment, the client is often directed to return to the front desk or billing area to remit payment in full (usually in the form of cash, check, or credit card) for the services rendered during the appointment. In addition to the current services received, the client may be given an estimate or charge proposal for future services, including anesthetic procedures.

It is imperative the veterinary practice collect payment from the patient at the time services are rendered and for the entire fee. This is critical to the management of the practice's accounts receivable. If the bill is collected at the time of service, there is never any impact on the accounts receivable balance. Only on rare occasions should patients be allowed to receive services that are not paid for immediately. An example is an emergency situation that generates a large bill a client may not immediately be able to pay. Payment for all routine and less urgent services should be collected immediately. If the client is allowed to leave without paying, the chance of collecting immediately decreases. Then the practice has to invest even more money in staffing to work the accounts receivable balances in an effort to collect for services rendered.

Although pet health insurance for veterinary medicine is not widespread, some clients may subscribe to it, and its popularity is expected to grow. Pet insurance is getting to be a big business, with U.S. premiums estimated at $275 million in 2008 and growing by 18 percent annually. There have been many developments in veterinary medicine, and these new options can get very expensive quickly. Pet health insurance helps people be able to say yes to those treatments.[1] However, unlike most forms of medical insurance, under these plans the client makes the entire payment due (usually at the point of service) and then submits applicable claims to the insurance company for reimbursement. Veterinary practices rarely deal directly with third-party payers such as insurance companies.

Another type of patient billing used occasionally is when the client elects to utilize a patient financing company such as CareCredit®, which extends short-term lines of credit for the payment of health services. The lender agrees to pay the veterinary practice in full at the point of service for any charges the client has incurred, minus a fee for this immediate and guaranteed payment. The client must then reconcile payment with the lending company independently, but the practice has already received payment.

Other Components of the Revenue Cycle

Maximizing revenue also involves other factors. The first is client credits and refunds. If a practice erroneously charges a client in excess of what was due, it must refund the difference to the client. These refunds must be documented carefully to ensure that the decrease in revenue is realized in the practice financials. Because the refund process is somewhat onerous, the practice should ensure that quality control mechanisms are in place so that payments are accurate and properly recorded, and refunds occur as infrequently as possible.

Another important component of the revenue cycle is staff investment. Employees of a veterinary practice must receive proper education in all facets of the revenue cycle and their role in its success. Employees should be invested in the establishment of policies and procedures that help maximize revenue. They should be asked to demonstrate current knowledge of the key components of the revenue cycle at regular intervals. Although few practices actually do this, a great initiative is for a practice to provide rewards (fiscal and otherwise) to employees whose productivity and performance assist in the generation of revenue. With employees involved in every step of the revenue cycle, it is important that they grasp the importance of their role and that the practice support them in any way necessary.

Key Revenue Indices

Because revenue in a veterinary practice is almost solely derived from client payments, the key revenue indices are the charges captured and the corresponding collection of these charges. First, a practice should evaluate its charges in terms of overall patient volume and the cost per service. Does the total patient volume correlate with the total amount of charges? What is the average charge per encounter? Are there certain procedures for which charges are not commensurate with the work performed? Should certain services or medications be charged at a higher rate because of the staff needed to perform the service or the time and materials needed to complete it? Answers to these questions will help determine whether or not the fee schedule used by the practice is appropriate, which is exceedingly important.

Next, the practice must consider its collections. What is the total practice revenue? What are the collections per veterinarian? Dividing total practice revenue by the number of full-time equivalent (FTE) veterinarians on staff can help evaluate productivity against the level of revenue currently being generated. The practice management software generally provides these data.

STEPS TO ENSURE REVENUE MAXIMIZATION

There are four key steps to making sure that revenue is maximized in a veterinary practice. Each should be completed on a routine basis to ensure the continued financial success of the practice.

Step 1: Analyze the Practice's Revenue Cycle

Consider the entire revenue cycle, from appointment scheduling through receipt of payment for any service rendered or good purchased. It is important to analyze each component individually and in concert with the other factors to determine where inefficiencies exist and where duplications can be eliminated. Improving each of the stages of the revenue cycle has the potential to increase revenue, which should be an overarching goal for any practice, and provides a definitive reason why revenue cycle analysis should occur regularly.

Step 2: Document Financial Policies and Procedures

Having written documentation that carefully explains the practice's financial policies and procedures is an important proactive measure that will ultimately benefit its fiscal health. Proper documentation provides the vehicle for standardization of the policies that are intended to streamline the revenue cycle. A lack of standard policies can lead to confusion for clients and employees alike and potentially lead to conflict. For example, if a newly hired employee is unaware of the policies and procedures about the collection of payments at the point of service, the practice could stand to lose revenue that it has earned. Likewise, clients who are unaware of the collection policy may be unprepared to remit payment when they come in for appointments. The result is a delay in revenue or a potential loss of revenue, which could have been avoided through documentation of policies and employee and client education. To mitigate these risks, a veterinary practice should clearly define in writing all financial policies and distribute this information to all appropriate parties. One effective mechanism for notifying clients is to have a "new patient" form that clients fill out the first time they visit the practice. Clients must review the practice's financial policies and procedures and sign to acknowledge their understanding of and compliance with these issues before patients are seen for their first appointment. Another effective mechanism is to post signs explaining the policies and procedures in the lobby, waiting areas, and treatment rooms.

Step 3: Review the Financial Tools

Whether a practice uses paper or software to document the treatments administered during a patient visit, the forms used to record the services must be straightforward and easy to use. If a veterinarian cannot enter the codes to generate the charges, the revenue cycle is in jeopardy. Likewise, if billing personnel cannot understand the coding form or the billing entry system, the revenue cycle is at risk. The tools that staff and veterinarians use to generate and capture revenue should be assessed for clarity, comprehensiveness, and appropriateness to the practice. If employees see ways to improve these tools, their ideas should be heard and discussed. A tool might work for its primary user, but to truly be of value, it must work for all users.

Step 4: Review the Practice's Current Fee Schedule

As mentioned previously, a practice's fee schedule is an important component of the revenue cycle. Many practices struggle in determining whether their fee schedules are appropriate. The fee schedule should be analyzed on a regular basis (at least once per year, but preferably several times throughout the year) to ensure that it accurately reflects the services and work being delivered and the cost to the practice of providing these goods and services. For example, as the costs of supplies, pharmaceuticals, rent, technology, and staffing increase, the fee scheduled should be modified to reflect these increases. Most often the price charged for the various products (medical and nonmedical) that the practice sells are adjusted as the cost the practice incurs to procure them fluctuates. Most of these products are "marked up" from their cost to determine the sales price the practice will charge. For example, a product purchased by the practice for $20 might receive a 50 percent markup to a sales price of $30. Should the price the practice pays for the product increase to $25, the practice might be inclined to increase the sales price to $37.50 to maintain the 50 percent markup. This process can become tedious if the practice markets a large number of products. However, appropriate emphasis should be placed on managing the retail prices of products to ensure that the practice maximizes profitability from these sales. Inattention to product pricing could result in the practice selling products for little profit and even at a loss.

The fee schedule for services should also be reviewed regularly to ensure that the prices reflect the market value of those services and allow for the desired profit margin.

Practices should be aware of the Consumer Price Index (CPI) and should increase prices annually, at a minimum, to be in line with changes in the "cost of living." Best practices go well beyond simply adjusting the fee schedule for services annually based on cost of living changes; they include quarterly reviews of the fee schedule to ensure the rates charged are (1) in line with what the market dictates and (2) ensure the practice is profitable to the extent desired by the practice owners.

REVENUE ENHANCEMENT

In addition to conducting regular reviews to ensure revenue maximization through improvements in the revenue cycle, there are other ways to enhance revenue. For example, a review of veterinarian productivity should also be performed at least once per year (perhaps in conjunction with annual performance reviews) to determine which procedures the veterinarian performs most often, which ones he or she performs least (or not at all), and what his or her production is in terms of total annual volume and average daily volume. This evaluation should occur on a monthly basis for veterinarians who are paid using a productivity model. Productivity-based compensation takes a variety of forms, but the most common is for a veterinarian to be paid a percentage of his or her monthly productivity in addition to a small base salary. The veterinarian's productivity can then be compared with the previous year's numbers for incentive reasons and performance reviews. In general, productivity can be compared with historical performance or benchmarked against other veterinarians in the practice. The practice may also choose to reward veterinarians for meeting specific productivity goals. As veterinarians' productivity increases, so will revenue, and the practice should consider providing incentives for veterinarians for the positive effect their increased productivity has on the practice as a whole.

Another way to enhance revenue is by growing the practice. This can occur as a result of adding a service line or offering a specialty service, expanding into a facility that allows greater capacity, establishing another location, or increasing the number of veterinarians in the practice. It is important to note, however, that although each of these actions has the potential to increase revenue, new capital or overhead costs are associated with all of them. A cost-benefit analysis should be completed prior to any of these undertakings to ensure that it will benefit the practice financially.

A simple way to increase practice revenue is to perform patient follow-up to boost client compliance. Often a veterinarian will recommend a certain number of treatments to deal with a specific ailment. The client frequently does not follow through with all of the recommended treatments, which may hinder the health of the patient and also decreases the potential revenue from the recommended treatment plan. Implementing a strategy to follow up with clients to ensure, to the extent possible, that they are following through with the recommended treatment plan could have a substantial impact on increasing revenue. The AAHA conducted a compliance study in 2003 and a follow-up study in 2009 to find ways to increase compliance. The results of the initial study have been published in *The Path to High-Quality Care*, and those of the follow-up study have been published in *Compliance: Taking Quality Care to the Next Level*.

SOURCES OF REVENUE

Here are the most common sources of revenue available to a typical veterinary practice:

- Patient encounters
- Surgical procedures
- Vaccinations
- Dentistry
- Diagnostic examinations
- Boarding
- Ancillary services (including laboratory, microchip ID, radiology, and ultrasound)
- Pharmacy
- Retail sales (including dietary products, flea and tick products, and shampoos)

To understand the overall financial benefit from each source of revenue, the practice should perform routine service line financial analyses, which involve calculating and evaluating the income that is achieved from each revenue center against the costs incurred to generate that level of revenue. With that information, the practice can then identify its most profitable areas, where potential growth can occur, and which service lines could be eliminated should their revenue not outweigh their overall cost.

To ensure that this analysis is as beneficial as possible, it must be completed with an accurate matching of revenues and expenses within each revenue center. This is pivotal because whereas one revenue center may generate a smaller amount of income, the limited expenses incurred to generate that income may result in a higher profit margin than another revenue center that generates a large amount of revenue but has a high level of expenditures associated with it, thereby limiting its profit margin. The practice may decide to maintain both of these service lines, but without completing this type of financial analysis, decision makers will not have adequate information on which to base their conclusion.

PRODUCTIVITY DEFINED

In previous sections of this chapter, productivity-based assessment of veterinarians and staff in a practice was highlighted as essential to comprehensive revenue cycle management. However, before these assessments can be conducted, productivity itself must be defined. Following are the most encompassing productivity measures in a veterinary practice.

- Encounters/visits
- Procedures
- Surgical procedures
- Consultations
- Charges
- Payments
- Ancillary service procedures
- Ancillary service revenue

Each of these measures defines productivity differently, yet each is relevant. For example, encounters are one way to account for a veterinarian's time and efforts. However, if a veterinarian has many encounters but does no procedures, is he or she productive? In terms of encounters, the answer would have to be yes, because the veterinarian's volume is high, but in terms of revenue, the answer would be no, because he or she is not performing any treatments that will ultimately generate revenue. When using productivity-based assessments, it is important that the measure be aligned with the overall goals of the practice. For example, if the practice wants to increase the number of patients seen per day, then counting visits would be an appropriate measure. If a practice wants to increase its revenue, then measuring procedures, charges, or payments would be more appropriate than adding up the number of encounters. Although a veterinarian's productivity can be assessed using many different metrics, it is important that these metrics be well understood, well documented, and in alignment with the practice's overall goals.

ANCILLARY SERVICES

Like other medical practices, a veterinary practice has the opportunity to provide ancillary services for its patients. Examples of traditional ancillary services are grooming, boarding, and product sales, both medical and nonmedical. These services, which go beyond basic clinical well-being, allow practices to earn additional revenue and meet clients' personal and convenience needs. Although some of these services result in only a meager profit, many practices decide to provide these amenities because clients request them, and ensuring client satisfaction is one of the ways a practice helps to guarantee a steady revenue stream. Although veterinarians debate whether offering products and services of this nature compromises the professionalism of veterinary care, and some believe that veterinarians should stick to providing medical care only, others disagree. Many clients appreciate the convenience of one-stop shopping for pet products and services.

SUMMARY

The generation of revenue allows a veterinary practice to continue to serve the needs of its clients and patients while also helping to meet its financial obligations. A practice's revenue can be maximized by adhering to the principles of revenue cycle management. These guidelines allow a practice to capture and collect all appropriate fees for the services and goods they provide. If a practice does not commit to diligent and consistent revenue cycle management, it stands to lose at least a portion of the revenue that it has rightfully earned.

Note

1. Steve Jordon, "Buffett Company Offers Health Insurance for Pets," *North Platte Telegraph,* October 8, 2009. Available at http://www.nptelegraph.com/articles/2009/10/08/news/ state/60004282.txt. Accessed October 14, 2009.

CHAPTER 3

Controlling Expenses

Veterinary practices should be continually mindful of costs and expense controls. Maintaining overhead (another term for the general expenses, or cost, of running a business) must be at the forefront of any successful veterinary practice. Both owners and employees should consistently focus on limiting costs to have a viable business in the long term.

This chapter focuses on a review of expenses, with particular emphasis on their control. Although veterinary practices present their expenses in various ways, Chapter 1 emphasizes that all overhead expenses should be part of the overall control strategy. Sometimes the veterinarians' expenses and the expenses of other individuals who generate revenue, their costs in salaries and benefits, will be stated in a separate section of the income statement. Other expenses, such as those illustrated in Table 1.1, include all salaries and benefits within the overall overhead of the practice. Whatever is the preference for presentation, without exception these important components of practice expenses should be determined, consistently presented, and managed.

The objective of this chapter is to consider the best strategies for controlling and maintaining overhead at an acceptable level.

EXPENSE MANAGEMENT

As in most businesses, veterinary expenses are simply divided into major classifications or descriptions (i.e., *accounts*). These may vary from day-to-day operational costs, such as salaries and benefits of staff, to repairs and maintenance, to supply purchases, and to longer-term recognition of costs, such as depreciation, amortization, and interest on debt. How detailed should the individual expense line items on the income statement be? There is no right or wrong answer to this; however, most successful managers are able to retrieve and, in turn, review in the income statement a fairly detailed listing of expense line items. It is important to note, though, that too much detail can render an income statement worthless. Through trial and error, a practice should determine the right amount of detail. The income statement should provide an appropriate level of detail to make informed observations and decisions, but not so much that every single dollar being spent is scrutinized. A good gauge of the appropriate level of detail on an income statement for a small practice should be that, when printed, it comprises no more than one or two pages. Also see Chapter 4 for more information on assessing financial performance, both from an expense and a revenue perspective.

Comparison of expenses on a line-by-line basis is also an important part of financial analysis and expense control. For example, the income statement illustrated in Table 1.1 presented both the current year and the prior year on a comparative basis. Taking this one step further, Table 3.1 shows the same income statement with several significant components added. The first is a column beside each line-item dollar amount that illustrates each line item as a percentage of total revenue. Sometimes this is called *right sizing* or *common sizing*; the expenses are illustrated as a percentage of revenue. Another column has been added to show the variance in both dollars and percentage differential between the prior and current years' numbers. This variance should be used to make a quick analysis, documenting the reasons for significant changes on both an absolute dollar and a percentage basis.

Table 3.1 illustrates one preferred way for the profit and loss statement to be presented, and in particular for expenses to be monitored; that is, a direct comparison with the prior year on a line-by-line basis with percentage differentials. Two other methods of comparison are (1) with the budgeted totals (again on a line-by-line basis) similar to the comparison to the prior year and (2) with industry standard benchmarks.

Comparing expenses with budget is a most important tool for controlling expenses. Comparing with the prior year is likewise important, yet changes may occur from one year to another that make such comparisons invalid. Comparing the budgeted totals always calls for a complete "apples-to-apples" comparison. If something significant has changed during the course of the year in accordance with the veterinary practice's accounting policies, the budget could be adjusted to reflect the change. For example, six months into the year, one of the veterinarians in the practice leaves, taking away much of the business. This change has a major effect on both revenue and expenses, until the practice has time to adjust by adding a new veterinarian. In this instance, it would be entirely appropriate to adjust the budget to reflect the change. Chapter 7 discusses in detail the whole budgeting and "pro forma" process. (Pro formas are another way to describe the effect of projecting operating results through financial modeling.)

TABLE 3.1

Example of an Income Statement (Modified Cash Basis)

ABC VETERINARY ASSOCIATES, P.A.
Statement of Income and Expenses for the Years Ended December 31, 20XX and 20XX
See Accountant's Compilation Report

	Year 1 (20XX)	% Sales	Year 2 (20XX)	% Sales	Increase/ Decrease	% Change
INCOME						
Veterinary Services and Sales	$ 1,053,343	100.00%	$ 915,950	100.00%	$ 137,393	15.00%
COST OF GOODS AND SERVICES						
Supplies—Medical and Resale	189,602	18.00%	164,871	18.00%	24,731	15.00%
Laboratory Fees	36,867	3.50%	32,058	3.50%	4,809	15.00%
Total Cost of Goods and Services	226,469	21.50%	196,929	21.50%	29,539	15.00%
GROSS PROFIT	$ 826,874	78.50%	$ 719,021	78.50%	$ 107,854	15.00%
EXPENSES						
Administrative						
Advertising	10,533	1.00%	9,160	1.00%	1,374	15.00%
Amortization	378	0.04%	329	0.04%	49	14.89%
Bank Charges and Processing Fees	17,907	1.70%	15,571	1.70%	2,336	15.00%
Contributions	2,100	0.20%	1,500	0.16%	600	40.00%
Dues and Subscriptions	1,438	0.14%	1,250	0.14%	188	15.04%
Miscellaneous	6,600	0.63%	5,769	0.63%	831	14.40%
Professional Services	17,250	1.64%	15,000	1.64%	2,250	15.00%
Supplies and Postage	15,800	1.50%	13,739	1.50%	2,061	15.00%
Taxes and Licenses	1,053	0.10%	916	0.10%	137	15.00%
Travel/Meals	1,980	0.19%	2,591	0.28%	611	23.58%
Total Administrative	75,040	7.12%	65,825	7.19%	9,215	14.00%
Compensation and Benefits						
Owner(s) Compensation	75,000	7.12%	75,000	8.19%	0	0.00%
Associate Compensation	119,425	11.34%	106,553	11.63%	12,872	12.08%
Staff Compensation	228,575	21.70%	192,350	21.00%	36,225	18.83%
Contract Labor	7,475	0.71%	6,500	0.71%	975	15.00%
Insurance	21,067	2.00%	18,319	2.00%	2,748	15.00%
Payroll Taxes	26,470	2.51%	23,016	2.51%	3,454	15.01%
Continuing Education	1,725	0.16%	1,500	0.16%	225	15.00%
Total Compensation and Benefits	479,737	45.54%	423,238	46.21%	56,499	13.35%
Facility						
Depreciation	37,867	3.59%	32,928	3.59%	4,939	15.00%
Equipment Rental	1,857	0.18%	1,615	0.18%	242	14.98%
Rent	63,000	5.98%	63,000	6.88%	0	0.00%
Repairs and Maintenance	15,800	1.50%	12,122	1.32%	3,678	30.34%
Telephone	7,935	0.75%	6,900	0.75%	1,035	15.00%
Utilities	8,427	0.80%	7,328	0.80%	1,099	15.00%
Total Facility	134,886	12.81%	123,893	13.53%	10,993	8.87%
Total Expenses	689,662	65.47%	612,955	66.92%	76,707	12.51%
OTHER INCOME/EXPENSE						
Interest Expense	74,995	7.12%	65,213	7.12%	9,782	15.00%
NET INCOME	$ 62,217	5.91%	$ 40,852	4.46%	$ 21,364	52.30%

It is essential to budget accurately. The budget is a plan for both revenue and expenses, but because expenses occupy by far the greatest number of line items in the veterinary practice, it is even more necessary when formulating the budget to make detailed considerations on a line-by-line basis. The budget comprises the profit plan for the practice.

Benchmarks are a valuable tool for controlling expenses and should be part of the veterinary practice's expense controls. Benchmarks are often misused when applied as the only standard. Although expenses should be controlled, every practice has its idiosyncrasies, and in some instances, benchmarks are not based on scientifically compiled data. Rather, they are an accumulation of data from myriad sources and practices and are not always adjusted for geographical, size, structure, and other variances. Even so, comparing against benchmarks can be a valid way to assess expenses, if they are realistic.

Common Sizing

Common sizing, as mentioned previously, is an important management tool. In common sizing, expenses are stated as a percentage of gross or net revenue or net collections, depending on the accounting basis being used (i.e., cash, modified cash, or accrual). Stating all expenses as a percentage of revenue allows for a consistent and easily identifiable measurement of performance, not only for the current period, but from year to year. On an accrual basis, expenses are compared with net revenue. On the cash basis (or even modified cash basis), expenses are compared with actual net dollars collected (i.e., revenue as stated on the income statement).

Common sizing is expressed in terms of percentages rather than absolute dollars. It provides insight into the practice's operations unlike any other; it is one thing to consider absolute dollars and their effect, but quite another to apply a percentage of revenue in the analysis. This means that if it is unclear whether an absolute dollar amount is high or low (depending on the size of the practice and other differentials within it), consistency in financial analysis can be easily applied through the common sizing process. When reviewing overhead, therefore, expenses stated as a percentage of revenue can easily be consistently analyzed, regardless of the size of the numbers or overall size of the practice.

Another way to look at this is to consider practice overhead in a total pie that includes revenue. The portion of the pie that is not concerned with operating overhead is left for the veterinary owners via compensation and benefits. Preferably, the pie shows no more than 70 to 80 percent expenses, leaving at least 20 to 30 percent for the owner veterinarians. Individual overhead expenses (i.e., the 70 to 80 percent) should be listed individually on the income statement and their percentage of revenue noted.

The sum of these expenses, in effect, would be the nonveterinarian overhead of the practice. All expenses and each element of revenue would then be illustrated as a percentage of total income, providing the utmost information available for managing costs.

Variance Analysis

Completion of a variance analysis, as mentioned previously, is a commonsense process, yet is seldom applied in the management of veterinary practices. It requires going through the simple process of comparing both absolute and percentage variances of revenue and expenses on the income statement. Usually the financial manager and practice owners will establish a specific policy for expense and revenue variances, which will trigger a more detailed analysis of why these variances have occurred.

As an example of a variance analysis, a practice has budgeted salary dollars for nonveterinarians at $25,000 per month and 15 percent of revenue collected. Actual results in any given month are $30,000 and 20 percent. Such variances (i.e., $5,000 in absolute terms and 5 percentage points) not only justify but also demand a more thorough and detailed review of why the increase occurred.

Early warning trends can be detected with this analysis. For example, the increased salary expense is due to unchecked overtime. Overtime worked and paid at time-and-a-half rates can add up very quickly, and the question is whether it was necessary. If the work was necessary, perhaps an additional full- or part-time employee should be added, thus avoiding the time-and-a-half rates. In many instances, overtime is worked simply because there is no approval process; that is, no one in management is really paying any attention. The overtime is worked and is paid at an additional rate, and before long, expenses are out of control.

The variance analysis utilizes the income statement as an active process to review costs and ensure that they are under control. By requiring documentation (i.e., an explanation of why the costs are higher than budgeted) or some other standard such as the prior year (or even both), it demands more accountability, more follow-up, and ultimately sustainability/viability of the practice.

The variance analysis, whether performed by the office manager, accountant, or even the owner veterinarian, is extremely valuable information that helps the owner learn more about the financial management of the business and understand the causes of expense variances. Moreover, it forces research into the reasons for such significant changes in expenses, requiring explanations and ultimately action. It is an extremely valuable tool to ensure expense control in the practice. Needless to say, the sooner excess expenses are discovered, the easier it is to control them. Such early warning signals are invaluable in controlling expenses over the course of the year, yet they require the process (i.e., the variance analysis) to be done every month to ensure that any excessive costs are investigated. (As a side note, the variance analysis should also consider significant *under*budget expenses. This could signal where not enough resources are being dedicated to a particular initiative, resulting in less revenue and overall return on investment, too.)

In summary, the variance analysis supports the trite but true statement that "we cannot fix what we don't know." If the practice doesn't know an expense is either high or low compared with the budget, the prior year, or some other standard, it cannot correct the matter.

TYPES OF EXPENSES

To review the expenses of a practice, it is best to break them down into major classifications. There are two major ways to review expenses: the overall category of expense and whether the expense is direct or indirect.

Overall Expense Categories

The basic expenses are grouped into four major classifications:
- Fixed expenses—those that remain stable/unchanged, regardless of volume
- Variable expenses—those that will change and be directly influenced by volume
- Semivariable expenses—those that vary within ranges of volume
- Semifixed expenses—those that remain stable or unchanged within a particular range of volume, then increase incrementally

For the most part, these four classifications can be divided between fixed and variable, with those that are between the two being the semivariable or semifixed costs.

Fixed costs are the easiest to manage because they do not change and should remain the same, at least throughout the course of the year. Rent, professional liability insurance, depreciation on furniture and equipment, and to some extent personnel costs are examples of fixed expenses. Personnel expenses are an area in which an expense could be both semivariable and semifixed, depending on the specific status of the employee. For example, it could be semivariable if the employee is on a fixed salary but also gets a bonus that is tied to production. The latter component of that compensation calculation would be semivariable. A personnel cost that is semifixed would be the base salary on an hourly rate, with overtime being paid at a higher rate. This is because the employee worked over the normal allotted time and was paid extra via the overtime.

In veterinary practices, variable costs typically represent a large portion of the practice's total expenses. This is because of the inventory costs associated with product sales. In many cases, inventory/product costs are the second highest expense, after personnel. A variety of costs could be considered variable, but inventory is clearly the main variable cost.

Although fixed expenses clearly make up the majority of the practice's overhead and are the easiest to control (because they do not change), they have both good and bad characteristics from an overhead control standpoint. The good news is that they do not change with revenue and are stable from month to month. The bad news is that they are more difficult to reduce because they are stable from month to month and often tied to a working relationship through employment or a contractual relationship such as a lease agreement.

Variable expenses should be tied directly to the production of revenue; therefore, as revenue goes up (or down), variable costs should do likewise. For example, the cost of pharmaceuticals administered to patients would likely vary with the volume. Sometimes, however, these variable costs can be controlled simply by the amount of inventory that is carried. For instance, the key to controlling variable expenses is to maintain as low an inventory as possible, yet to maintain sufficient quantities to serve the needs of the patients. This balance is very important because inventory levels and supply purchases can have a large impact on the financial performance of a practice. For example, if too much inventory is purchased at a time, cash flow management may be difficult. Alternatively, if the practice does not maintain enough inventory, providing services to patients may be difficult. It is therefore important to be aware of how inventory is used and the demand for certain products. This includes identifying seasonal and other trends that may influence the need for certain items. Inventory should be managed on a regular basis to ensure that purchases are of appropriate size and frequency. This will help to smooth out the practice's earnings and manage cash flow. This is especially true for those practices that use the cash basis of accounting because, as discussed previously, they effectively expense the cost of supplies when they are purchased.

Figure 3.1, a cost-volume-profit graph, shows the four types of expenses within overall expense. Basically, this graph points out that in every veterinary practice, a certain number of patients or a certain volume must be reached (or amount of work must be completed) to attain a break-even point. Once the fixed costs are covered, the only additional expenses for all intents and purposes are variable. Further, because the variable expenses are significantly lower than the fixed costs, the practice becomes marginally more profitable with each additional patient or unit of revenue realized.

Every veterinary practice has a point in time (i.e., day, week, month, or year) when it reaches a break-even point, when the fixed costs have been covered or fully absorbed

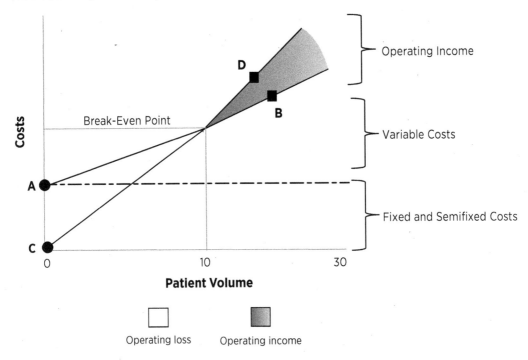

FIGURE 3.1
Cost-Volume-Profit Graph

ABC Veterinary Associates, P.A.

A = Fixed Costs + Semifixed Costs, represented by ▬▬ ▬ ▬▬ ▬ ▬
Fixed Costs and Semifixed Costs include Rent, Staff, Utilities, Malpractice Insurance, Information Systems, Furniture/Equipment.

B = Total Costs (Variable + Fixed at 25 patients per day, for example)
Variable Costs include Administrative Supplies, Medical Supplies, Pharmaceutical Supplies.

C = Revenue at 0 patients seen

D = Revenue at 20 patients per day

and the only additional costs are the variable expenses. Because the variable expenses are much lower, once the break-even point is achieved, the profit of the practice (i.e., the monies that are left to be distributed to the owner/veterinarian) will increase. Hence, in Figure 3.1 the shaded area of operating income gets larger as the volume (i.e., the dotted horizontal line) increases.

To apply the theory shown in Figure 3.1 to real-world practice, the opportunities for increasing revenue and the bottom line are most practically stated by simply increasing the number of encounters per day, week, month, and year. As the encounters are plotted (i.e., the dotted horizontal line in Figure 3.1) on the graph, the practice generates greater operating margins. Another way of saying this is that the most profitable patient each day is the *last one*. Once the fixed costs are covered in any given period, all other encounters are more profitable because only variable expenses are left to be absorbed.

When considering the total overhead of the veterinary practice (especially when separating the veterinarian compensation and benefits into a different classification of overhead, similar to the income statement illustrated previously in this chapter), it is obvious that most expenses are fixed or at least mostly fixed. Therefore fixed costs must be managed carefully. They are best managed by controlling them before they are incurred. In other words, staff should not be added before it is reasonably certain that revenue will be increasing. Likewise, the practice should not launch out too broadly into increased space and higher rent without some assurance that the revenue opportunities will improve.

Direct and Indirect Expenses

As mentioned previously, another way of looking at expenses is to categorize them as direct and indirect. Direct expenses are those that can be traced to a specific medical service provided (e.g., salary expense, supplies, materials used directly to perform the service). Indirect expenses are those that cannot be traced to a specific service (e.g., billing, utilities, accounting, rent). The importance of separating direct and indirect expenses lies in both the ability to assess performance within various profit or cost centers where such allocations are made and the overall ability to control these expenses. Direct expenses are usually more controllable because they relate directly to income production. In the veterinary practice, the boarding component would have certain direct costs, such as the rent for the space being used for those services and the staff who are specifically assigned to such services. With these expenses directly allocated against that profit center of revenue, they are easily identifiable and more easily managed. Indirect expenses are usually more complex because they are the result of a somewhat arbitrary allocation process. Indirect expenses must be allocated to the various profit centers based on what should be a consistent set of assumptions applied across the entire practice. For example, billing and collection of services is a "corporate" expense that is done centrally and is a support service for all of the profit centers in the practice. Thus, the cost of the staff, facilities, supplies, and so on (i.e., both fixed and variable costs) would be allocated in some fair and equitable manner among all of the various profit centers. It is important to note that certain expense categories, such as staff and supplies, could represent both an indirect and a direct expense. As an example, support personnel working in the boarding department would be a direct expense to that department, but support personnel working in accounting would be considered an indirect expense to the boarding department as well as other areas.

Although the allocation of indirect expenses is extremely subjective, if done consistently it provides great integrity to the financial statements. Moreover, it enables management to make good decisions based on the performance of each individual profit center, which is the primary objective. This detailed level of accounting is not performed in most veterinary practices because of the level of complexity involved. The cost of having an accounting department perform these allocations outweighs the benefit of the additional information it provides, especially for smaller veterinary practices. Nevertheless, this level of accounting makes sense for a large practice that encompasses multiple providers and has numerous profit centers generating substantial revenues. The detailed accounting may be more useful for small practices when occasionally performing an analysis of a specific profit center. In these instances, it may make sense to go through the process of allocating some indirect expenses to better understand the true profitability of the profit center, but not as an ongoing process. The bottom line is that, when it comes to this type of financial analysis, each practice must determine the level of detail needed to effectively manage that practice. In no way should detailed accounting become so cumbersome that it distracts the veterinarian from normal duties, which are to see patients and generate revenue.

Thus, direct and indirect expenses are a major factor in the overall overhead and cost considerations (i.e., controlling expenses) of the veterinary practice. Being able to break down and allocate expenses—either on a direct basis into each profit center or on an indirect basis to a varied number of profit centers—allows the practice ownership and/or management to be more effective in assessing and evaluating performance. The ability to control expenses is undoubtedly enhanced.

MAJOR CLASSIFICATIONS OF EXPENSES

The veterinary practice has major classifications of overhead that should be considered as part of the overall strategy for presentation of the financial statements, and even more important, for enabling the practice to achieve greater control of the costs. These major classifications are as follows:

- Compensation and benefits
- General and administrative
- Facility
- Cost of goods sold (supplies, laboratory, etc.)
- Veterinarian compensation and benefits

Figure 3.2 illustrates the relationship of these major classifications of overhead, but with owner compensation included in the compensation and benefits section and interest expenses as its own section to represent the "Other Income/Expenses" category shown in Table 1.1. In some cases, a practice will split out owner compensation and nonowner veterinarian compensation, so that it can see all of its overhead other than veterinarian compensation and benefits and show its operating profit prior to this expenditure. When this is the case, the costs of veterinarian benefits, salaries, bonuses, and so on are classified and illustrated separately on the financial statements. This could be broken down further into owner and nonowner veterinarians. Nonowner veterinarians could be a subclassification of expenses within the total veterinarian salary and benefits section. This is strictly up to the individual practice, but can provide more insightful information for the owners to determine what compensation is "left over" for them. That final amount may be distributed 100 percent as compensation, or a portion of it may be retained in the business as equity (i.e., retained earnings).

The following discussion considers these five major classifications of expense and how they may best be controlled. These five expense areas are important for segmenting total overhead of the typical practice. Although it is essential to know the contents of the individual line-item expense of each major classification, a broader perspective

FIGURE 3.2

Expenses and Overhead

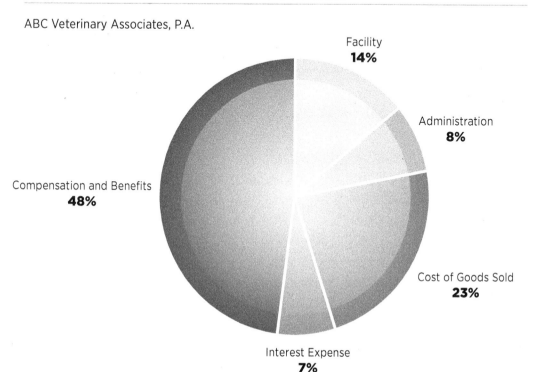

ABC Veterinary Associates, P.A.

Facility **14%**

Administration **8%**

Compensation and Benefits **48%**

Cost of Goods Sold **23%**

Interest Expense **7%**

on each of the major classifications will help the practice owner/operator control costs on an overall basis.

Compensation and Benefits

The largest single expense in most service businesses, including the veterinary practice, is personnel. This encompasses all expenses attributable to staffing. It is important to note that veterinarian compensation and benefits are not typically separated in most veterinary practices' financial statements because of the wide use of QuickBooks™ as their accounting software, which does not easily allow for this customization. However, most practices do list owner compensation and associate veterinarian compensation as separate line items on their income statement. Veterinarian compensation and benefits are discussed later in this chapter, with the understanding that from a presentation standpoint they are often joined with all other compensation and benefits.

All personnel costs, including clinical support associates, administrative associates, and other staff, should be considered within this broad classification. When all these costs are accumulated, this is the greatest area of practice expense. This is true regardless of design, history, subspecialty, and services provided.

The number of staff should be measured within the framework of each individual practice. One of the greatest challenges for any business (including a veterinary practice) is how many employees are needed. This question is often the most difficult both to answer and to substantiate; how large a staff is necessary to provide quality and responsive service without overspending and adding significant dollars to the bottom line? The typical veterinary practice should have nonveterinarian staff expenses that are roughly 20 to 30 percent of collected revenue; clearly, staff numbers require strict control.

A key approach to controlling personnel costs is to consistently monitor workflow and emphasize cross-training. The skill mix of the staff is also important. In some cases, for example, it may seem easier and better from an economic standpoint to hire a less experienced associate. However, because of the additional training and lack of efficiency of that individual, it may be preferable to hire a more experienced person who costs more but provides greater efficiency and a higher return on investment.

The ideal scenario is to hire a balanced skill set. The objective is to employ a combination of experienced individuals who will stay with the practice over the long term, building up greater salaries and benefits, while providing more efficient and customer-responsive performance. At the same time, less skilled and less experienced individuals who cost less to employ are always needed. To achieve the right balance, one strategy is to blend employees with different skills and experience levels. Through training and development, including cross-training, these employees will increase their ability to handle greater responsibilities and enable more experienced individuals to perform at higher levels of efficiency.

Another possible scenario for cost containment is outsourcing. Typically, practices limit outsourcing to specific departmental functions such as administrative oversight, perhaps the accounting and billing/collections work. Usually outsourcing entails greater direct costs yet is not necessarily less efficient, depending on the available skill set and the practice's history of staff turnover.

Another strategy in controlling personnel expenditures is engaging in independent contractor relationships. In a way, using independent contractors is another form of outsourcing, although the veterinarian can work virtually full-time (within certain IRS and legal parameters) yet not be paid as an employee. Independent contractors are paid only when they actually work and are not guaranteed a fixed salary each month. Generally, independent contractors do not get benefits, which results in significant savings to the practice. The downside is that contractors are free to work or not, which can be detrimental to practice performance. The upside is that this is an excellent way to manage costs from month to month as practice volumes ebb and flow. The IRS has specific criteria for what constitutes an employee versus an independent contractor. Accordingly, should a practice choose to contract with veterinarians rather than employing them, it will be essential to confer with a tax accountant to ensure that the contractual relationship established will stand up to IRS scrutiny. Furthermore, it is important to keep in mind that if a practice chooses to contract with veterinarians as opposed to employing them, the compensation rates will often be higher because the contracted veterinarian has to pay self-employed payroll taxes, insurance, and other personal business expenses.

Independent contractors are not the same as "relief doctors" used to fill a temporary need. A relief doctor is more akin to a *locum tenens* in the health-care industry. Essentially this is a doctor who has no previous relationship to the practice and is simply brought in to provide services during another provider's absence. For example, if a veterinarian suddenly went on medical leave, a relief doctor might be brought in to provide continuity of service.

Like most service businesses, veterinary practices have peaks and valleys in staffing needs throughout the day and week. When monitoring personnel costs, it is best if the veterinarians keep busy throughout the normal workday, with appropriate support staff available. Some (although not many) practices use veterinary time equivalents (VTEs) to measure the overhead being passed on to clients. This is a means of measuring the time a veterinarian spends providing services. The overhead cost, when measured, is spread over the time availability of those individuals who generate professional fees and other revenue, namely, veterinarians, technicians, and assistants. In some instances, this allows the practice to calculate and measure overhead on a per-minute basis, depending on the level of staffing required and the length of the procedure being performed. Although most veterinary staff members are busy throughout the normal workday and workweek, it is difficult (if not impossible) for every minute of the day to be billable to one client or another. The many nonbillable activities include communication with staff and clients as well as mundane projects such as cleaning and research to prepare for, or after seeing, a particular patient, when such research and preparation cannot be billed to the client. Within a given workday, typically only half the time is directly billable to specific clients.

Another use of VTEs is to apportion personnel costs for any given procedure, based on staffing parameters and the time required to complete the procedure. For example, if a per-minute billing rate is determined for veterinarians in the practice (often $4–$6 per minute at current production metrics), the cost of the support staff is usually a fractional total of this amount. Technicians, for example, are compensated at about one-third of the amount of the associate veterinarian, and assistants to the veterinarians are typically compensated at about one-fourth of the veterinarian's cost. Thus, when looking at staffing, it is most appropriate to provide a balance of optimum cost that also provides appropriate support to the veterinarians.

Figure 3.3 summarizes major staffing strategies. These strategies are applicable to every component of the veterinary practice and, if followed, may lead to a stronger bottom line.

General and Administrative Expenses

The veterinary practice should monitor all costs of a somewhat general nature. Often these are referred to as general and administrative (G&A) costs. Predictably, they encompass a variety of individual line items, such as the following:

- Maintenance and repairs
- Dues, subscriptions, and licenses
- Janitorial and custodial expenses
- Postage and freight
- Accounting and legal expenses
- Gifts and contributions
- Other professional services

G&A expenses encompass a broad cross section that includes many important components of support for the practice. From a cost control standpoint, these expenses

FIGURE 3.3
Major Staffing Strategies

ABC Veterinary Associates, P.A.

1 Increase volume

- Patient encounters
- Procedures
- Ancillary services

2 Increase number of providers served per full-time-equivalent staff

- Apply realism

3 Review systems to identify inefficiencies

- Eliminate tasks/steps
- Minimize exceptions

4 Evaluate staff skill mix

- Review credentials
- Evaluate skill sets

5 Minimize turnover

- Identify critical performance measurements
- Hire staff with multitask skills
- Cross-train after employment
- Create stable environment
- Use predictably consistent management structure
- Reward performance
- Include incentive pay

6 Remove incompetent staff

- Use a legal and professional approach

7 Provide adequate staff training

- Conduct regular training at all levels

8 Ensure that personnel and compliance policies are written and followed

- Perform self-audit and periodic independent reviews

9 Establish realistic salary ranges for practice positions

- Be competitive and consistent

are not usually significant when viewed individually. For example, the total of account-ing expenses, which usually encompasses support for the practice's accounting on a month-to-month basis plus quarterly and annual tax preparation, in and of itself is not a significant amount, usually well under 1 percent of total revenue. Yet when this expense and the others classified as G&A are consolidated, they comprise a significant portion of the total overhead—perhaps as much as 15 percent of the overhead and 10 percent or more of revenue.

These expenses are largely controllable because in many instances they are attribut-able to services provided by outside suppliers or professionals. Further, some are based at least in part on an individual decision by the owner about the level of cost. Items such as dues and subscriptions, for example, are somewhat arbitrary, not necessary, expenses. Other expenses, such as janitorial and custodial costs, may be limited based on the will of the owners to do some of that work themselves (usually such work would be done after hours). This approach has its downside, as the staff members are generally paid overtime to do this work, and they often resent such tasks and the extended hours. Time spent doing patient work makes much more sense than covering janitorial services.

To control G&A expenses, it is best that the practice owners have a line-item bud-get for each such expenditure. Monitoring these budgeted amounts on a regular (i.e., monthly) basis is extremely important. Also, because most of these costs emanate from an outside vendor and are supported by either a contract or an invoice, these docu-ments should be reviewed and approved prior to paying bills.

Another way to control expenses is to assign one individual, such as the practice (or office) manager, the responsibility for purchasing and vendor selection. This indi-vidual should be given specific guidelines and protocols for purchasing, with a fixed dollar amount as a ceiling for authorization. Moreover, periodically the practice own-ers should review purchasing activities to make sure no special deals are taking place. Sometimes vendors will take practices for granted, and a service or its price will not remain competitive. All suppliers should undergo comparative competitive reviews.

G&A expenses are a key item to monitor within every component of the practice's operations. In and of themselves, these costs may be relatively minor, yet they are not insignificant for the overall practice. Moreover, because they recur, it is essential to support them with strong controls and approval processes, including a line-item bud-geted total.

Facility

The cost of the facility is the rent or mortgage payment plus other direct expenses at-tributable to the use of the space, such as utilities. Most veterinary facilities are owned by the practice owners (i.e., usually the veterinarians) or by another legal entity that is owned by the same individuals (i.e., the veterinarian owners of the practice), then leased to the practice. The cost of the facility is in essence tied to the cost of the building and the resulting debt service or imputed debt service that would result. If the facility is leased from a totally independent party, that lease amount should be negotiated in good faith, based on market rates and whether the practice can afford and justify the expense of the specific space.

Another major component of the facility cost is the build-out, sometimes referred to as tenant improvements to the facilities. These can vary depending on whether the space is complete when it is first procured. If the lease is taken out when the structure is basically a shell (i.e., nothing is finished), the cost of the tenant improvements will be significant and is merely another component of the total rental amount. This cost may be passed through to the lessee practice via rent. Or, based on the negotiated settlement relative to the lease, the tenant improvement costs may be expended by the practice, with that interest and debt service being the effective facility cost on an ongoing basis.

Most leases are negotiated on a fixed basis, which does not allow a great deal of flexibility. In other words, the cost negotiated is essentially set for at least a year, with most veterinary practices having multiyear leases. Therefore, the control of this cost is accomplished by maximizing revenue, or perhaps if not all the space is needed, by subleasing a part of it to other related services. Another way to control facility costs is to make the best use of the space by converting as much of it as possible into revenue-producing space. For example, excess space could be converted into additional boarding area to provide the practice with more capacity for boarding pets overnight, on weekends, and for extended periods. This is a great source of revenue, and the revenue generated may more than offset the cost of the space.

Utilities are another major component of facility expense. Utilities vary with use but can be controlled through monitoring the use of electricity, water, and gas, as well as developing efficiencies for controlling consumption.

Thus facility costs, though fixed, can be controlled (at least as a percentage of revenue) through maintaining higher revenue and through space utilization (i.e., shifting as much "dead" space to revenue-generating square footage as possible).

Cost of Goods Sold

Clinical supplies and related costs pertaining to the production of revenue are an ongoing expense that is a major part of the overall practice operations. These expenditures are mostly variable because they change with revenue. The more patients are seen and procedures are performed, the greater the number of supplies that are consumed. However, these costs can be controlled through maintaining optimal levels of inventory, keeping as little as possible on hand so that the cost of inventorying supplies is only temporary. This would also include such things as radiology expenses, even though the cost of the radiology equipment itself would be mostly a fixed expense. The supplies that support that equipment would be variable, analogous to other clinical supply inventories.

Although cost of goods sold is a variable cost that will be greater in absolute dollars with more revenue (which is the hope in all practices), it should be possible to maintain it as a percentage of revenue at a relatively predictable level, especially if inventories of the supplies are controlled. When the practice performs accounting on a cash basis, all supply items are expensed when they are purchased and paid for. Thus, the amount of inventory is irrelevant in terms of a costing factor because it is all expensed at the time it is paid. Because many (if not most) veterinary practices use cash-based accounting, the need to control inventory is obvious. But this is also the case for practices that use accrual-based accounting, because even though the cost of unused supplies is carried on the balance sheet, it is a drain on cash flow and ultimately will also be an expense to the practice on the P&L statement.

Veterinarian Compensation and Benefits

The single largest expense for the practice should be the veterinarians themselves. In many instances, one or more of these individuals will be the owner of the practice. Compensation for the nonowner veterinarians should be considered part of the overall expense management of the practice. As previously outlined, this classification of expenses can be presented separately so it is relatively easy to distinguish the nonveterinarian overhead from the veterinarian overhead. In most cases, the owner veterinarian's compensation is twofold. First, he or she is typically paid a specific salary that is in line with market levels, just as nonowner veterinarians are paid. The owner veterinarian also receives any income/profits generated by the practice as additional compensation. This is illustrated in Table 3.1. Of course, it is the owner's decision whether to leave any profits in the practice to fund future growth or take the profits as compensation. Furthermore, the method by which the profits are paid as compensation can vary based on what type of legal entity the practice is. For example, in C corporations, the profits of the practice to be paid as compensation are typically paid out as a bonus, which is considered additional expense to the practice, so as to avoid taxation at the corporate level. In an S corporation, the profits of the practice to be paid as compensation may be paid out as a bonus or treated as a draw on the owner's equity in the practice. Most often, the practice's tax accountant provides guidance in this area about which method makes the most sense from a tax perspective.

Nonveterinarian employees typically do not have the mindset of an owner or a professional who is trained to provide most of the highly technical services. However, the associate veterinarians (those employed by the practice) have a greater stake in the business, even the possibility of becoming an owner partner in the future. Therefore, it is important to establish specific compensation guidelines that promote responsiveness on the part of the associate veterinarians (i.e., give them incentive to think like an owner), as in any professional entity where associates may aspire to become part of the ownership.

The first step to creating an equitable and effective compensation plan for the employed veterinarians is to target pay levels for each position, perhaps tied to tenure or performance. (In reality, this should also be the process for developing the compensation structure for all other employees—only the pay scales are lower.) Not surprisingly, the compensation structure for the associate veterinarians should be a combination of both straight (guaranteed) salaries and incentives for additional compensation, normally tied to personal production. Measuring job performance is extremely critical in every case, which is often best done through individual productivity, assuming the volume of work is available for that individual. Also, associate veterinarians are compensated as a percentage of their production. The compensation could be totally at risk or, as noted above, a combination of straight or guaranteed salary plus a percentage of production after certain thresholds of collected productivity are achieved. Moreover, this could be tiered at different levels, with the percentage going up after attaining each respective threshold.

The compensation system for owner veterinarians is obviously different from that for associates, as they are more likely to be compensated explicitly for their management results (i.e., the profit they produce). In a practice with several partners, production could encompass various responsibilities for each partner.

Factors that influence an associate veterinarian's salary are related to the economic performance of the practice, which must be a major part of the compensation structure. However, market rates must also be considered, as well as the credentials and experience of the associate veterinarian. Once these specifics are incorporated, the compensation structure should be determined and instituted through a well-defined compensation plan. The plan should include the incentives as well as the base pay. Benefits are also a major part of compensation, and their economic value (i.e., cost to the practice) should be part of the compensation analysis and the overall structure. Many veterinary practices (and other small businesses) enter into contracts with their employed veterinarians simply through a handshake. The handshake arrangement comes with much risk, as there is no binding agreement with which to hold both parties accountable. Accordingly, it is best practice to have a written employment agreement or professional services agreement with every employed veterinarian. Furthermore, it is important to ensure that these contracts are current and clearly state the existing arrangement between the provider and practice. Although legal counsel will be needed to draft and update contracts, the cost is usually minor.

No compensation model is perfect; however, the ability of associate veterinarians to realize additional income through greater productivity is a major positive factor that in most cases will produce a win-win scenario. The practice benefits through greater productivity, and the employed veterinarian benefits through receiving additional compensation. That said, straight salaries also have some value, in that the doctor is compensated for all work, not just the medical/surgical production. All must spend time in management and administrative functions, including training and supervising employees, meeting with suppliers, and marketing the practice. All of this could be covered by a straight salary. Conversely, the advantage to tying at least a portion of the salary to production is that the incentive is there to reach out and complete more medical/surgical encounters. In this context, the administrative, marketing, and other indirect productivity functions should be considered part of that guaranteed or base salary.

Conceivably the best compensation structure provides both incentives for the day-to-day functions of a veterinarian (with some not tied to productivity) and incentives that are directly tied to productivity. Productivity bonuses that are tied to a percentage of production for medical/surgical services, along with a fixed salary for the other activities, appear to offer that win-win formula that works best. Bonuses should be established that are neither too easy nor too difficult to attain, for example, bonuses that start with certain levels of production or after those levels of production are sufficient to cover the base salary from the standpoint of return on investment. Thus, when production reaches the level where the bonus is applicable, the ownership of the practice is also benefiting from that excess percentage. Typically the normal production percentage is in the neighborhood of 20 to 22 percent, which may be tiered. That is, when higher levels of production are attained, the percentage can creep upward.

One critical component of a veterinary practice that cannot be overlooked is the need to ensure the delivery of quality clinical care. In some instances, when a productivity model is in place, a veterinarian may "overutilize" in an effort to be more productive, to the extent that quality suffers. To ensure that this does not occur, it is important to provide proper oversight of the veterinarians and perhaps build some quality measures into the compensation model.

The compensation structure for owner veterinarians is tied to overall practice performance. Typically, owners are compensated at a guaranteed fixed amount, with additional bonuses effectively tied to the profit of the organization. Likewise, veterinarian owners may have tiered levels of compensation, with tiers tied to personal production and management responsibilities, and the final tier being the bottom line of the practice.

This part of veterinary practice expenses is an integral part of the overall management of the practice. Veterinarian compensation—for both owner and associate, as well as their benefits—will be the single largest expense of veterinary practice; therefore, it must be continuously managed and monitored.

Incentive Strategies

A final component of the expense structure is incentive strategies. Although these may apply to both nonveterinarian and veterinarian employees, they should be a major consideration in the overall overhead structure. Incentive compensation is a proven value to employees as well as veterinarians. Giving all employees the opportunity for additional incentives through compensation, benefits, and time off is a demonstrated way to motivate higher levels of performance and output. The incentives do not constitute a great financial cost to the practice; nevertheless, they are relevant in terms of total compensation to each employee. They should be significant enough to make a difference in behavior and overall actions.

SUMMARY

Managing overhead is a major part of the practice owner's responsibilities. In some instances, the focus on revenue production is overemphasized, while expense management is overlooked. When management of expenses is neglected through lack of expense or overhead control, profits can suffer dramatically. The methods of breaking down the expenses by components discussed in this chapter are a major way to better understand, manage, and control costs. Monitoring expense performance on a day-to-day basis, from the source level of approval, such as the invoice or purchase order, to the presentation of the financial statement, is essential to achieving success in the veterinary practice.

CHAPTER 4

Assessing Financial Performance

One way for a veterinary practice to measure its financial performance is by keeping a close watch on the balances in its bank accounts. As long as money is available, it can be spent, and the practice may be assumed to be doing well. When the money runs low, expenses must be reduced or additional income generated. Although this approach to financial management may appear comical to most people (and for good reason), it was the method used by many veterinary practices for a long time; in fact, some small practices are still managed this way. However, the use of this process is becoming more difficult to justify as it is proven unsuccessful in one practice after another. The problem with this method is that available money is not the only indicator of a practice's financial health, and it does not convey what changes need to be made to improve performance.

This chapter addresses how financial performance must be diligently managed using a comprehensive analysis of a practice's assets, liabilities, revenues, and expenses. Assessing financial performance does not mean just taking note of the changes in numbers on monthly financial statements. Rather, assessing financial performance should be thought of as an intensive and ongoing process necessary to help a practice maximize its potential for success. Only when a practice uses quantitative analysis of financial performance to drive decisions is it truly managing its financial health. Although we have touched on many of these methods of financial analysis in previous chapters, this chapter covers them in greater detail and describes when you would use one method versus another.

FIRSTHAND ANALYSIS OF FINANCIAL PERFORMANCE

Setting up financial statements should be the first step a practice takes in its assessment of financial performance. Once the structure for each of the major financial statements has been created and the appropriate categories are listed in each, the practice must populate (either manually or preferably through an electronic resource) the statements with the appropriate data and run summary reports at least once per month. These reports are then analyzed to determine the practice's current financial performance, including improvements that have taken place and changes that need to be made. If a practice does not use its past financial performance to help make meaningful decisions for the future, the financial statements are essentially only as useful as the "balance in a bank account method" described above.

Table 4.1 illustrates opportunities that can be seen when analyzing financial statements and the actions that may be taken to capitalize on these opportunities.

THE EFFECT OF ANALYZING FINANCIAL STATEMENTS
ON LONG-TERM FINANCIAL MANAGEMENT ISSUES

Though all financial statements correspond with a certain time period, their useful life far exceeds the time period they represent. It is imperative that a veterinary practice use financial statements in its strategic planning and long-term decision making, because current financial performance will likely affect how a practice chooses to spend or save in the future. Long-term strategies such as buying new equipment, adding another service line, adding another veterinarian, moving or adding locations, and remodeling existing facilities need to be considered well in advance, as appropriate capital or cash reserves must be built up in preparation for these expenditures. For example, technology is becoming more widely used in the field of veterinary medicine, and even small practices are beginning to compete with specialty practices by acquiring the advanced equipment needed to perform various tests and procedures such as ultrasounds, laser surgeries, and digital radiographs. However, how will a practice know if it has enough money reserved for a major equipment purchase if it does not know what its historical and current money levels are? The only way to determine that is by using the financial statements.

When considering long-term strategies, it is important to assess the impact from both a revenue and an expense viewpoint. For example, if a practice wants to add a new veterinarian, what are the possible revenue benefits and costs associated with that additional employee? It is important to consider the effects of that addition beyond just the revenue the veterinarian will produce and the cost of salary and benefits. Once the veterinarian is hired, will improvements to the facility be necessary to create a usable working space for that person? What are the costs for additional

TABLE 4.1

Opportunities from Analyzing Financial Statements and Actions to Capitalize on Them

Opportunity 1: Revenue is decreasing.
Action Items
- Review charge capture, billing, and collection process to ensure it still effectively meets the needs of the practice.
- Adjust the fee schedule.
- Review productivity by provider to see where decreases are occurring.
- Have management review practice internal controls to ensure their effectiveness.
- Review practice internal controls with employees to ensure compliance.
- Review provider status.
  - » Are greater amounts of provider PTO being taken?
- Does the current staffing model provide appropriate coverage?
- Assess work and office hours.
  - » Are the practice's office hours still meeting current and potential clients' needs?

Opportunity 2: Staff salaries are high and increasing.
Action Items
- Consider realigning the existing staff.
- Place a moratorium on wage increases.
- Consider the use of a productivity-based compensation program (where applicable).
- Consider the use of an incentive pay program, wherein some portion of an employee's total compensation is held at risk.
- Eliminate overtime.

Opportunity 3: Drug and supply costs are higher than projected.
Action Items
- Review current buying process.
- Review existing vendor contracts (as applicable).
- Research group purchasing organizations.
- Consider switching drug supply/office supply companies.
- Review current inventory; consider keeping less inventory on hand.
- Assess the security of supplies; consider moving them to a more restricted location if necessary.

supplies and equipment that will be used by that veterinarian? Will additional staff members (front-office staff, veterinary technicians, etc.) also have to be hired to maximize the new veterinarian's productivity? Newly hired veterinarians often take more than a full year to ramp up their operations to the point where their productivity is commensurate with other, more established veterinarians. Can the practice financially support that veterinarian until a more developed revenue stream is produced? Also, when new veterinarians are added, the remaining veterinarians may realize a transient decrease in their productivity as clients are now being shifted among a greater number of veterinarians. Will the practice be able to support these veterinarians in the interim as well? These questions should be analyzed and answered in depth; one way to do so effectively is to complete a cost-benefit analysis for each strategy long before it is implemented, quantifying the current costs, the incremental costs associated with the strategy's implementation, and the financial benefits that will be realized after implementation. With this analysis, the practice will be able to determine if the benefits of undertaking a new initiative will outweigh the costs, and therefore whether or not the strategy should be considered further.

Financial statements have been developed so as to have predictive value or feedback value. If the statements are not used with those purposes in mind, they are of very little value to a practice. Therefore, it is important that a practice treat financial statements as more than a sequence of numbers and use them as an integral tool in the economic decision-making process in both the short and the long term.

OTHER INDICATORS TO WATCH

Of course, it is essential to review the key financial statements (balance sheet, income statement, and statement of cash flows) each month, but it is also important to consider other indicators, such as these:

- Number of visits
- Number of new clients seen
- Revenue from clinical services
- Revenue from pharmacy sales
- Revenue from ancillary services (broken down by service line)
- Revenue by veterinarian (differentiated between employed veterinarians and owners)
- Average charge per encounter (in total and by veterinarian)
- Accuracy of the front-desk staff in billing and collecting payment
- Pharmaceutical/drug costs (both in real dollar terms and as a percentage of total revenue)
- Other supply costs (broken down by clinical and office expenses, and expressed in real dollar terms and as a percentage of revenue)
- Veterinarian compensation expense (both in real dollar terms and as a percentge of revenue)
- Staff salary expense (both in real dollar terms and as a percentage of revenue)
- Ancillary service costs (broken down by service line and presented in both real dollar terms and as a percentage of revenue)
- Rental expense (including facility and equipment rentals, expressed in real dollar terms and as a percentage of revenue)

- Net income before owner compensation
- Net income after owner compensation
- Cash on hand at the end of the month

This list may seem too lengthy to be vetted on a monthly basis, but it is only by considering each of these metrics that accurate financial planning and informed decision making can occur. Data relevant to each of these metrics should be compiled by the middle of the following month, and the results should be compared with the previous month and the same month in the previous year (e.g., January of Year 1 compared with January of Year 2). Most veterinary medicine software programs used in everyday practice have a report module that allows for searching and reporting a variety of variables. As discussed further in Chapter 10, the key is to utilize the software to the fullest and continue to upgrade it as necessary so that it may be used in assessing financial performance with ease and clarity.

The following additional indicators should be considered routinely, although these may be considered on a bimonthly basis:

- Clinical staffing per full-time-equivalent (FTE) veterinarian
- Administrative staff per FTE
- Employee turnover rates
- Number and total amount of client refunds
- Appointment availability
- Patient wait times (presented separately for patients with an appointment and those who access the practice on a walk-in basis)
- Patient cancellation/no-show rate
- Veterinarian cancellation rate
- Number of referrals

These factors do not require as diligent a review as those discussed previously, yet they are important and should be considered regularly as part of the financial assessment of the practice.

MEASURES OF PRODUCTIVITY

As discussed in Chapter 2, there are many different measures of productivity in a veterinary practice, including charges, collections, patient visits, procedures, and consultations. Each offers a different lens through which to examine veterinarian and total practice productivity. However, these measures should not be considered in a vacuum, completely independent of each other and without context. It is important that a practice analyze productivity in total and by veterinarian each month. The current level of productivity should be compared with previous months to determine if a trend is developing. As positive trends arise, the practice owner or manager should determine their root cause and decide whether or not the driving force behind the trend can be used to positively influence other areas in the organization. For example, practice managers notice that revenue is increasing month over month. When this is investigated further, it is determined that the cause for this increase is that one veterinarian has been steadily increasing her patient encounters and procedures. When asked, the veterinarian states that she has been putting forth more effort because of the practice's new productivity-based compensation incentive, which rewards her for achieving a set threshold of encounters and completed procedures per month. The practice, realizing the benefits of a productivity-based incentive program, may then consider using this sort of program with other veterinarians and modifying it to include nonclinical staff members as well.

VARIANCE ANALYSIS

The difference between an actual and a projected value is called *variance*. As part of the ongoing financial assessment of a practice, variance analyses should be conducted regularly to highlight areas where projections were not realized and why the discrepancy occurred. When conducting a variance analysis, actual values on an income statement are compared against specific standards derived from budgeting, profit plan totals, industry benchmarks, or even prior month (or prior year) revenue or expense totals. Although not every line item in the income statement will be considered in depth, those items that vary significantly from their corresponding standard should be analyzed in greater detail. The results of the variance analysis should then be used to consider where and why there are differences between actual and budgeted financial performance, whether or not any variances are part of an ongoing trend, and what actions can be taken to rectify (or continue) the variance going forward. The variance analysis is yet another instrument in the financial assessment toolbox and should be used to help make corrections and adjustments in a practice to ensure its continued financial well-being.

Tables in previous chapters presented examples of income statements (see Tables 1.1 and 3.1), with Table 3.1 showing an example of a variance analysis completed for a veterinary practice's combined statement of revenues and expenses (i.e., income statement). This statement is presented for a year-over-year variance analysis, but a similar analysis could just as easily be completed for a month-over-month period or some other period. Because these examples were illustrated in prior chapters, there is no reason to include them again here. However, it goes without saying that use of a combined revenue and expense statement is a great means of assessing the financial performance of the practice.

BALANCE SHEET CONSIDERATIONS

The income statement is likely the most commonly used financial tool; however, the balance sheet complements and adds to the information depicted in an income statement. As discussed in Chapter 1, the balance sheet provides information about a practice's assets, liabilities, and owners' equity at a specific time. The balance sheet provides all the information needed to create and manage the accounting equation (Assets = Liabilities + Owners' Equity). Although the balance sheet can be more confusing to practice managers than an income statement (particularly for individuals without developed business and financial acumen), it is important that this financial statement be prepared accurately and reviewed regularly. If a practice is unable to generate a full balance sheet from its accounting system, it may be able to pull some of the balance sheet data from the system, and should do so regularly. If the practice uses an outside accountant to prepare the balance sheets, it should ask to receive a copy monthly. If a practice receives only one balance sheet per year, it is capturing only the accounting activity on that single day. Without balance sheets from previous periods, the practice will have no way to compare its current financial standing against prior performance. Such a financial statement would have limited use.

ROLE OF OUTSIDE PROFESSIONALS

Accountants, CPAs, consultants, tax advisors, attorneys, and financial planners are all weapons in a veterinary practice's financial assessment arsenal. These outside experts offer knowledge not held by any member of a practice's staff and are particularly useful during the following life cycles of a practice:
- Prior to creation of a legal business entity
- Prior to opening the practice for operations
- When creating and managing a practice's financial statements
- Prior to merging with another practice or other business entity
- Prior to acquiring another practice or other business entity
- When determining the practice's fair market value
- Before adding or contracting with additional veterinarians
- During tax season (and beyond)
- Before making any large capital expenditures
- When looking to improve work process flow
- When mitigating personnel issues

Although an outside professional may be engaged at any time by the practice, some professionals should be used on an ongoing basis. For example, an accountant should be used as an advisor throughout the year (especially if the practice prepares its own financial statements, which as discussed above, should be analyzed monthly). A tax advisor should also be consulted on a regular basis to ensure that appropriate planning for both short- and long-term tax liabilities is occurring.

When selecting an outside professional, it is important to choose a person or organization that fits the practice's needs. Ask managers in other local practices whom they use, and what their opinion is of that person or organization. Use the Internet to research prospective candidates. Another excellent resource for veterinarians is VetPartners (www.vetpartners.org), a veterinarian-specific, not-for-profit entity that provides resources and references to outside professionals who have specific experience in the

TABLE 4.2

Best Practices for Appropriate Tax Planning

Goal: Decrease taxable income.

Action Items

- Project business and personal earnings for a three-year period to prepare for all applicable tax brackets (at higher incomes, different rates of taxation are possible).
- Take advantage of legal tax deductions, including those related to travel, automobile use and meals, and entertainment expenses.
- Postpone year-end billings, dividend distribution, and the sale of property or investments that produce a capital gain until the next tax year if you expect your tax rate to be lower at that time. Conversely, accelerate these payments if you think your tax rate will be higher in the next tax year.

Goal: Maximize safe harbors for tax payments.

Action Items

- Use designated safe harbors to avoid penalties for late tax payments or underpayments (payments are generally due January 15, April 15, June 15, and September 15 of each year).

Goal: Reduce marginal tax rates.

Action Items

- Gift investments to children, who are assessed at a much lower tax rate.
- If a sole proprietor, consider hiring your children as employees, thus exempting you from FICA, Medicare, and unemployment taxes.
- Structure income transactions so that they are subject to capital gains, which are generally taxed at a lower rate.
- Select the practice's legal entity with care (C corporations and partnerships often receive the least tax benefits).

Goal: Maximize tax credits.

Action Items

- Setup and fund tax-deferred retirement programs, such as 401k and IRA, which provide the practice with tax credit for the amount it contributes.
- Claim construction costs that improve access for disabled persons (made legal under the ADA).

veterinary industry. When you have selected a few possibilities, call them directly and ask for a list of their references. Take the time to call those references and hear what they have to say. Consult the licensing board for the applicable industry and ask for a list of certified professionals in your area. While you are selecting an outside professional, be open and honest with potential candidates about your needs and expectations for fees, deliverables, and timelines. Ask for documentation or a written agreement that describes the services that will be provided, and review it carefully before signing.

Tax Considerations

There are many forms of taxation applicable to a veterinary practice. Of course tax evasion is illegal, but the process of tax planning can help a practice to minimize, defer, or eliminate certain taxes. It is often advisable for a practice to contract with an outside tax accountant to ensure that appropriate tax planning and preparation occur and the practice remains compliant with any federal, state, or local guidelines. Table 4.2 provides a list of goals and action items related to tax planning.

SUMMARY

The overall success of a veterinary practice is determined by its financial performance. It is impossible to gauge the success of a practice without having a full understanding of the practice's financials. Financial statements such as the balance sheet, income statement, and statement of cash flows are the tools used to assess historical and current performance. These statements are best utilized for their predictive or feedback value, meaning that their real benefit lies in their ability to determine future performance or highlight areas that are either profitable or require improvement. Financial statements are designed to assist in economic decision making in both the short and the long term; when practices use them this way, they will be better prepared for the future.

CHAPTER 5

Ratios and Benchmarking

As we've seen, an important aspect of the ongoing management of the veterinary practice is analyzing financial data. This means not just briefly reviewing balance sheet and income statements on a monthly basis, but also examining the data and performing calculations to understand the practice's inner workings from a financial perspective. Analyzing the financial statements of the practice is more than just looking at the balance sheet to make sure there is cash in the bank and then looking at the income statement to ensure the practice is generating a profit.

This chapter explores two components very important to thorough financial analysis: ratios and benchmarks. Calculating certain financial ratios and comparing the business with industry benchmarks are more detailed methods of determining performance. Done properly and consistently, they can quickly provide determinants of financial performance, allowing practice managers and/or owners to fully understand what is occurring in their practice and to make any necessary changes.

RATIOS

In simple terms, ratios are a means of testing relationships, that is, comparing one financial figure with another. In the financial sense, ratios are comparisons of performance measurements from the two major financial statements, the income statement and the balance sheet. Additionally, ratios are used to analyze operational data, such as the number of patients per FTE (full-time-equivalent) veterinarian. These two primary ratio uses can also commingle; for example, it is often beneficial to use an operational figure and compare it with a financial figure. An instance of this is calculating the average transaction per patient. This would involve using the number of patients the veterinary practice serves for a certain period as well as the revenue generated during that same period.

Although an unlimited number of ratios can be derived, most businesses use specific ones on a consistent basis to monitor their performance. Some are applied to the general business arena, whereas others are specific to veterinary practices. The discussion below explores a number of the key ratios that will be beneficial to managers and owners of veterinary practices when considering the financial performance of their business.

Key Ratios

This chapter discusses key ratios that veterinary practices should consider. This discussion is by no means all-encompassing, as there are several others that can be considered. In fact, many practices take the basic ratios discussed in this chapter and tailor them to their specific needs to provide the most useful information. Furthermore, many of these ratios can be applied in various ways. For instance, they can be used company-wide or on a more departmental basis, to examine how certain service lines contribute to the overall financial performance of the practice. The following sections illustrate these key ratios in more depth and explain how they may be applied in a veterinary practice.

Revenue and Profitability Ratios

A number of ratios can be used to focus on the veterinary practice's revenue and profitability. These measure primarily how profitable the practice is and its progress in collecting or generating revenue. Some of these key ratios are listed below and then further considered throughout this section.

- Net profit margin
- Gross profit margin
- Average transaction charge
- Revenue per FTE veterinarian
- Accounts receivable

Net Profit Margin

A very common ratio for any business is the net profit margin ratio. Essentially, this divides the profit of the business by the revenue generated:

$$\frac{\text{Practice Profit}}{\text{Practice Revenue}} = \text{Net Profit Margin}$$

Most businesses use a bottom-line approach in this ratio, wherein all expenses are considered in deriving the profit to use in the calculation. For veterinary practices, there are two alternatives: using the profit *after* veterinarian compensation and benefits are subtracted and using the profit *before* veterinarian compensation and benefits are subtracted. The distinction is important because they can generate very different results.

In many instances, the veterinarians are the sole owners of the practice, and therefore any profit generated belongs to them. It is up to the owners whether this money is paid entirely as compensation or some is left in the practice to fund future growth. Accordingly, in this instance the true profit of the practice is what is generated before the owners are paid; thus, calculating the profit margin using profit before veterinarian compensation likely makes the most sense.

In other situations the veterinarians are not the owners of the practice and are paid a salary just like any other employee. In these circumstances, it makes the most sense to calculate the profit margin using profit after all veterinarian compensation and benefits. This will show a lower profit margin, but is reflective of the true profit of the business to the owners. Other factors to take into consideration when calculating a profit margin are those outlined in earlier chapters relative to true profitability. This includes the depreciation taken on various assets, the rental rate charged to the practice (should the owners of the practice also own the real estate), and other discretionary expenses that are related to the owners of the practice. You can find a profitability estimator at www.ncvei. org, the Web site of the National Comission on Veterinary Economic Issues (NCVEI).

The profit margin ratio can be calculated for the entire practice or for particular business units. For example, if the practice provides kennel boarding services, it could analyze the profitability of this particular service line.

When analyzing the profit margin, a higher value is always better, as this means that more of the revenue generated falls to the bottom line and is not consumed by the costs necessary to operate the practice.

Gross Profit Margin

Whereas the net profit margin looks at the overall profit of the practice compared with sales, the gross profit margin looks more specifically at how much it costs to make a product or provide a service. In a veterinary practice, this can be used to examine either the entire practice or a small subsection. Many practices are involved in product sales, such as pharmaceuticals or pet supplies. The practice must purchase these items, expending cash, with the intent that the products will sell for more than their cost. The difference between the cost of the product and the revenue it generates for the practice is the gross margin. For example, let's say there is a drug that costs the practice $65 per unit, but the selling price is $100 per unit. The gross margin would be $35 or, stated as a percentage, 35 percent. The gross profit margin formula can be illustrated as follows:

$$\frac{\text{Gross Profit}}{\text{Revenue}} = \text{Gross Profit Margin}$$

This measure allows a practice to analyze the products it sells to determine which are profitable. It is important to remember that the gross profit margin is prior to all other operating expense the practice incurs. Along the same lines, gross profit may be calculated for the provision of services by subtracting the cost of providing services (i.e., veterinarian and direct support staff time) from the revenue generated by providing that service.

Average Transaction Charge

The average transaction charge is an important ratio that allows a practice to understand exactly how much revenue is generated on a per transaction or patient basis. Having this information allows practices to analyze their patient patterns, the services they offer, and how the services are priced to determine whether changes should be made. Furthermore, this ratio can be tracked from period to period to identify issues in the performance of the practice. For example, if the average transaction charge decreases substantially in one month, it could signal that further analyses are necessary to understand the reason for the decrease. This formula can be stated as follows:

$$\frac{\text{Practice Revenue}}{\text{Practice Transactions}} = \text{Average Transaction Charge}$$

When calculating this ratio, it is important to remember that the revenue and transaction data should be for the same time period. For instance, if the revenue for the first quarter is being used, transaction data for the first quarter should also be used. A lack of consistency between the numerator and denominator will produce a result that has no meaning.

A positive trend would be the average transaction charge continually increasing. This would reflect that overall, the practice is able to generate the same amount of revenue from fewer transactions. Emphasizing product sales is a good way to increase the average revenue per patient.

Revenue per FTE Veterinarian

It is important to consider the productivity of the veterinarians, as they ultimately control the success of the practice. Accordingly, revenue should be measured on a per FTE veterinarian basis. This can be calculated using the following formula:

$$\frac{\text{Practice Revenue}}{\text{FTE Veterinarians}} = \text{Revenue per FTE Veterinarian}$$

If the veterinary practice's management system software tracks revenue specific to each veterinarian, this information can be compared using this ratio to monitor the performance of each veterinarian. Those whose performance falls below the average calculated should be told that improvement in performance is necessary. This information can also be compared against industry standards through benchmarking, described in more detail later in this chapter.

Accounts Receivable

Many veterinary practices operate on a strictly cash basis, requiring payment at the time services are provided, but others do not. They build up an accounts receivable balance, indicating the money they are owed from clients for services rendered. Just as with revenue and profitability, the accounts receivable balance must be analyzed to provide insights into how well the practice is performing. The most common methods of analyzing accounts receivable use two ratios, the accounts receivable turnover and the days in accounts receivable ratio.

An analysis of the *accounts receivable turnover* provides information on how many times the accounts receivable balance is converted into cash during a specified period. In most instances, this ratio is calculated quarterly or annually. The calculation for this ratio follows:

$$\frac{\text{Credit Sales}}{\text{Average Accounts Receivable}} = \text{Accounts Receivable Turnover}$$

There are several important points to consider in performing this calculation in a veterinary practice. First, the sales or revenue figure should include only credit sales. That is, cash sales or cash revenue should be excluded. This is because these revenues have already been collected and never affected the accounts receivable. If these revenues are included, they will skew the calculation, making the result look better than it actually is. Second, the credit sales and average accounts receivable balance should be aligned. If the calculation is for a certain year, the credit sales should be reflective of the entire year, and the average accounts receivable should be calculated using the beginning and ending accounts receivable balances for that year. Thus, average accounts receivable should be calculated using the following formula:

$$\frac{\text{Beginning Accounts Receivable}}{2} = \text{Average}$$

A higher value for the accounts receivable turnover ratio is better, as it indicates the accounts receivable balance is converted into cash more often. If the value is low, the practice should analyze its collection efforts and possibly limit the amount of accounts receivable clients are allowed to carry or discontinue the process altogether.

The *days in accounts receivable* ratio is similar to the accounts receivable turnover ratio, but instead of indicating how many times the accounts receivable balance is converted to cash, it indicates how many days a client balance sits in accounts receivable before being collected. The following formula is used to determine the days in accounts receivable. In fact, the accounts receivable turnover ratio is needed to calculate this ratio.

$$\frac{\text{Number of Days in Period}}{\text{Accounts Receivable Turnover}} = \text{Days in Accounts Receivable}$$

As noted above, to calculate the days in accounts receivable, divide the number of days in the period being analyzed by the accounts receivable turnover ratio. For example, if you are looking at the entire year, the numerator would be 365, but for a quarter it would be 90 days.

To illustrate, let's say that the accounts receivable turnover ratio is 12 for a full year. Thus, to calculate the days in accounts receivable, divide 365 by 12 to arrive at 30.42. This indicates that accounts receivable turns over approximately 12 times each year, or every 30 days.

As another example of what can be learned from this ratio calculation, 30 days in accounts receivable as of today means it would take 30 days to collect this balance. This means that over the year, 30 days of working capital is required to maintain this practice's cash flow needs.

Expense Ratios

Monitoring revenue, profit, and accounts receivable through ratio analysis is extremely important in performing a detailed analysis of the practice's operations, but special attention should also be paid to the expenses incurred by the practice. These ratios group expenses in similar "buckets" and then consider them in relation to some measure of productivity or performance. In a veterinary practice, the following ratios are most useful:

- Expenses as a percentage of revenue
- Expenses per patient
- Expenses per FTE veterinarian

The following discussion examines each of these in more detail.

Expenses as a Percentage of Revenue

Considering expenses as a percentage of revenue is often referred to as a "common size analysis" (see also Chapter 3). This means that all expense categories are illustrated as a percentage of a base figure, in this case, revenues. As noted previously, instead of considering each individual expense line item, it is often beneficial to group certain expenses. Listed below are four useful categories in which expenses can be grouped, including more detailed expense categories that also fall into these groups.

Personnel	**Occupancy/ Facility**	**Variable/Cost of goods sold**	**Fixed/ Administrative**
Staff salaries	Rent	Medical supplies	All other costs
Payroll taxes	Utilities	Product costs/	
Benefits	Repairs and	inventory	
Temporary labor	maintenance		

Use of this ratio allows a better understanding of the trend of expenses in relation to the revenue the practice is generating. For example, if revenue remains stagnant, it would be expected that the above expense categories, and calculated ratios, would remain consistent year over year. However, if revenue increased only slightly, it would be reasonable to assume that variable costs would increase proportionately, with the other categories remaining relatively neutral, in that they are mainly fixed costs. Fixed costs do not change with increases/decreases in revenue, whereas variable costs change proportionally to the increase/decrease in revenue. If there are major swings in revenue, it would be reasonable to expect that all cost categories would experience sizable movement. This is because fixed costs are fixed only to a certain extent.

Following is an illustration of how personnel costs as a percentage of revenue would be calculated. All other expense as a percentage of revenue ratios would be calculated in a similar manner.

$$\frac{\text{Personnel Costs}}{\text{Practice Revenue}} = \text{Personnel Costs as a Percentage of Revenue}$$

Just as in the net profit margin ratio, when calculating personnel costs as a percentage of revenue, veterinarians may be either included or excluded. If the veterinarians are the owners of the practice, they should be excluded. However, if they do not own the practice, they should be included as personnel.

Expenses per Patient

The practice may calculate the expenses per patient in the same way that it calculates the revenue per patient. This makes it possible for the practice to monitor how well it controls patient expenses. This can be especially useful when comparing period with period. To a certain extent, as productivity increases, the expense per patient should decrease. This is because a large majority of costs are fixed and are incurred regardless of whether one patient or a hundred are seen. Of course, even the fixed costs increase once the practice is operating at full utilization. The expense per patient is calculated as follows:

$$\frac{\text{Practice Expenses}}{\text{Practice Patients}} = \text{Average Expenses per Patient}$$

Expenses per FTE Veterinarian

Expenses can also be stated on a per FTE veterinarian basis. This involves dividing total expenses by the number of FTE veterinarians in the practice, as shown in the following formula:

$$\frac{\text{Practice Expenses}}{\text{FTE Veterinarians}} = \text{Expenses per FTE Veterinarian}$$

This formula is not limited to looking at expenses in total; smaller subsets of expenses may also be considered. For example, personnel costs are an important expense category that could be considered on a per FTE veterinarian basis. If certain costs are tracked per veterinarian, this analysis can be expanded further to analyze how the costs incurred vary from veterinarian to veterinarian.

Key Credit Ratios

The ratios considered previously in this chapter are important to the ongoing financial analysis of the veterinary practice. There are also other ratios veterinary practices should calculate on a regular basis. Some entail the analysis of credit indicators and creditworthiness. Often veterinarians are unable to borrow capital without providing their own personal guarantee. This is an issue when the practice needs a new, expensive piece of equipment or the owners desire to expand their practice through adding a new veterinarian or expanding the facility. Good managers should help veterinarians real-ize that certain key credit indicators must be present in order for them to borrow, such as a practice's capability to retain earnings and not distribute all earnings to its owners. Not distributing all profits to the owners may appear to have a negative tax implica-tion, yet this is not necessarily so. For example, the net income from the practice that is taxed via a pass-through scenario (a Sub-S corporation, limited liability company, or partnership) can retain earnings by simply distributing enough monies for the owners to pay their individual income taxes at their respective rates, usually 40 percent or less.

When considering key credit indicator ratios, the net income of the business and/or retained earnings has a significant effect on the creditworthiness of the practice and the owners' subsequent ability to borrow money without providing personal guaran-tees. Following are key credit indicator ratios and target requirements that creditors examine:

- Debt service coverage
- Debt to capital
- Return on equity (current ratio)
- Days cash on hand

These ratios are examined in greater detail below.

Debt Service Coverage

This ratio provides insight on how well the practice covers (or could cover) its debt obligations. It uses the following formula:

$$\frac{\text{Net Operating Income (after Veterinarian Compensation)}}{\text{Principal and Interest Payments}} = \text{Debt Service Coverage}$$

Net operating income is typically prior to income taxes, depreciation, and interest expense. A debt service coverage ratio below 1.0 is not a good indicator, as it essentially means the company can cover less than 100 percent of the total debt service. Anything above 1.0 is considered a positive sign, with a ratio of 1.5 being most desirable.

Debt to Capital

This ratio considers the portion of debt as a percentage of total capital, which includes both debt and equity. The ratio is calculated using the following formula:

$$\frac{\text{Total Debt (Including Leases)}}{\text{Total Debt plus Total Equity}} = \text{Debt to Capital}$$

Considering the limited amount of equity that most veterinary practices maintain, this ratio tends to be high. For example, if equity is 0, this ratio would be 100 percent, meaning 100 percent of the capitalization is debt, with no equity. A higher debt-to-capital ratio can indicate that a company is highly leveraged and more likely to default on its debt obligations. Considering that most veterinary practices do not maintain much equity, a higher debt-to-capital ratio is considered normal, but too high a ratio could have negative consequences when trying to obtain additional financing.

Return on Equity

The return on equity ratio compares the practice's net income with equity using the following formula:

$$\frac{\text{Net Income}}{\text{Average Equity}} = \text{Return on Equity}$$

Average equity is calculated similarly to average accounts receivable, by dividing the beginning and ending period balances by 2. Once again, it is important to make sure the net income figure and the average equity figure are for the same periods. If not, the resulting ratio could be misleading.

This ratio will essentially indicate the amount of income generated in relation to the level of equity. A higher return-on-equity ratio is desired. The return-on-equity ratio can be calculated both before and after veterinarian compensation. If the veterinarians own the practice, it should most likely be calculated before compensation to be more meaningful.

Current Ratio

The current ratio is widely used to quickly shed light on the viability of an organization. It can easily be applied to the veterinary world. The formula used is as follows:

$$\frac{\text{Current Assets}}{\text{Current Liabilities}} = \text{Current Ratio}$$

This ratio illustrates an organization's liquidity by showing the level of liquid assets over liquid liabilities. Essentially, if the only current asset were cash and the only current liability were accounts payable, the ratio would indicate how well the practice's cash balance could cover its accounts payable balance. This is important because a low or negative current ratio may indicate that a company is illiquid and unhealthy. A high current ratio is preferred.

Days Cash on Hand

This ratio indicates how many days of overhead the current level of cash could cover. The formula is stated as follows:

$$\frac{Cash}{(\text{Annual Operating Expenses} \div 260 \text{ days})} = \text{Days Cash Balance}$$

Essentially, the current cash balance is divided by the average operating expense per working day. Working days are used as opposed to total days because these are the days the practice is actually operating. As a general rule, it is a good business practice to keep 20 to 30 days' worth of cash on hand to ensure liquidity issues do not arise.

Nonfinancial Ratios

All of the ratios discussed above involve the measurement of data on either the income statement or the balance sheet. However, the use of ratios is not limited to these scenarios. In a veterinary practice, ratios can be used to measure numerous other data. Some of these are discussed below.

FTE Staff to FTE Veterinarians

Because personnel is one of the largest costs for any business, especially a service business such as a veterinary practice, it is important to ensure that only the necessary number of staff are employed. This can be determined by examining the number of staff employed per veterinarian using the following calculation:

$$\frac{\text{FTE Staff}}{\text{FTE Veterinarians}} = \text{Staff per Veterinarians}$$

Although calculation of this ratio alone does not indicate whether the staffing level is too high or too low, it does allow for period-over-period monitoring of the staffing level to ensure consistency. Furthermore, if there is a veterinarian change (i.e., a veterinarian leaves or joins), calculation of this ratio will provide guidance about staffing needs to accommodate the change.

New Patients per FTE Veterinarian

In terms of monitoring whether a veterinarian's practice is "full," it is useful to calculate the number of new patients per FTE veterinarian using the following formula:

$$\frac{\text{New Patients}}{\text{FTE Veterinarians}} = \text{New Patients per FTE Veterinarian}$$

This allows for the monitoring of growth from period to period and provides insight on the mixture of new and recurring patients in the practice.

It is essential to delve more deeply into the financial performance of the practice than by occasionally glancing at the financial statements. Use of ratio analysis is a beneficial and informative method of doing this. Ratios that are accurately and consistently calculated and supplied to administration and the owners of the practice on a regular basis will enable decision makers to evaluate performance quickly and make changes as necessary.

In summary, ratios are critical to the successful management of the veterinary practice. They are quick and to the point, and what they reveal is very insightful. They should be used on a regular basis (at least monthly) by the manager or owner and should be based on unvarying criteria and consistently applied so that they maintain credibility.

In many cases it is beneficial for a practice to develop a "flash report" of key ratios as part of the management reporting process each month. This succinct report of ratios (usually one or two pages) will be very revealing, and with regular use could be one of the most important components of the financial analysis process.

BENCHMARKING THE VETERINARY PRACTICE

Benchmarks, statistical comparisons that form economic standards against which to compare the actual performance of a practice, are important for measuring the veterinary practice's performance. Benchmarks allow for gauging the practice against independent measures.

When used judiciously, benchmarks enable a good comparative analysis. In certain instances, benchmarks should be used as primary comparisons against actual performance and might even be part of the financial statement comparisons. AAHA has several publications about benchmarking that are useful tools when used correctly.

Benchmarks should be used conservatively, as they are not always scientifically calculated. They are compiled from various trustworthy sources but often are unscientific compilations of data. Furthermore, changes in the methodology of accumulating and reporting the benchmarks can influence the end result. Thus, it is important to understand how the data are accumulated. For example, most benchmark sources exclude outliers (i.e., data that are clearly not consistent with the rest of the reported data on both sides of the spectrum). This is beneficial because it enhances the usability of the data. If the method of excluding outliers is changed, however, it can influence the data that are ultimately reported. The key is to ensure that the data are gathered, filtered, and reported in a consistent manner from year to year. Often, if there is a change in the methodology of the survey company, it is for a good reason and likely enhances the usability of the data. It is important to understand any changes that have occurred, their impact on the benchmarks, and the ensuing impact on the use of those benchmarks.

Benchmarks will vary by type of practice, number of veterinarians, number of locations, geographic region, size of the group, and other factors. Benchmarking is an ongoing process that uses an independent standard to compare productivity, expenses, and certain quality measures. It is also a way to establish targeted performance and is a good business/management tool for monitoring results. Like most methods of financial analysis considered in this book, benchmarking allows for objective, measurable performance standards to be compared against actual practice performance as a way to pinpoint trends and receive early indications about a strength or weakness, an issue, or a needed improvement.

A key point is that benchmarking is the use of external sources to evaluate internal performance. Although it is important to measure performance against internal standards, such as the budget and the previous year's performance, it is also beneficial to use external standards. Otherwise, performance that seems good may merely be acceptable. Even if the performance is good, it is essential to compare it against external sources or standards in pursuit of experience and knowledge of the business. For benchmarking to be credible, the data must be comparative, which is usually the greatest challenge when benchmarking. For example, when benchmarking the practice's revenue, the comparison should be "apples to apples."

The following questions illustrate some of the problems that arise when using benchmarking comparisons:

- Is the external source defining revenue in the same manner in which revenue is captured in the practice (i.e., inclusion or exclusion of ancillary sources of revenue)?
- Does the external source comprise practices in the same geographical location or metropolitan status?
- Does the external source have a patient population similar to that of the practice (i.e., dogs and cats only or all animals)?
- Does the external source include practices that are similar in size?

Similar problems arise for expenses:

- Are the expenses inclusive of any veterinarian benefits or salaries?
- Are employed veterinarians' expenses included in overhead?

These are the basic problems that surface when a practice turns to external sources, and they demand close analysis and definition. Once this information has been acquired, numbers usually can be adjusted to reflect functional benchmarks for comparison.

It is essential to define benchmarking comparisons and to use them consistently. Some benchmarking data are easier to compare. For example, patient visits used as a measurement standard are typically consistently applied from practice to practice and therefore do not pose an issue of consistency.

Other standards for benchmarking comparisons are also more viable when using data such as number of full-time-equivalent employees and costs. It also helps to break the data into smaller components, such as total support staff cost and even accounts receivable (e.g., total accounts receivable dollars over a certain number of days, aging, etc.).

Benchmarking Patient Access

Patient access, of course, is key to the success of any veterinary practice, starting with the process of appointment scheduling and continuing through the actual visit, with financial success often measured by the length of the appointment and the fees generated. The following details should be considered when establishing a benchmarking comparison based on the access component of the practice:

- Total number of appointment slots per day
- Type of appointment slots
- New patient slots
- Appointment length

With these benchmarks, measuring "apples to apples" may be difficult. Practices differ somewhat, yet there should be many similarities. As an example, the length of appointments in comparison with industry benchmarks should help other veterinarians understand general expectations. A better understanding of what occurs throughout the industry in this area could lead to more efficient scheduling, allowing more access to veterinarians and the potential for increased revenues. Still, what is good or acceptable, though guided by the benchmarks, is largely based on practice preference. For instance, if a veterinarian is extremely focused on patient care or tends to handle more complex issues, the appointment lengths may be longer than the benchmark standard, but may be justified by the individual's practice style.

Benchmarking the Fee Schedule

A major factor in the generation of revenue is how the practice determines the price of its services. Although there is no set rule about how a practice should set its fee schedule, it only makes sense to set it in line with what others are charging in the market. If the fee schedule is set too low, the practice is missing out on potential revenue. If set too high, it is likely the practice will not be able to attract new patients.

Numerous benchmarking sources allow veterinary practices to compare their fee schedules against national and regional standards. This may be one of the most important types of benchmarking a practice can perform, as it is a "front end" and not a "back end" comparison. That is, the benchmarking process is performed prior to the revenue generation activities, as opposed to at the end of a financial period. Every practice should benchmark its own fee schedule at least annually to ensure it is charging market rates.

Accounts Receivable Benchmarks

Several key ratios reviewed in this chapter also can be used as benchmarking comparisons. Most sources that compile statistical data provide key accounts receivable indicators, such as days in accounts receivable and accounts receivable aging, in terms of outstanding balances (typically in 30-day buckets).

Moreover, these comparisons can be illustrated visually in ways that have a tremendously informative impact on the operation. In Figure 5.1, for example, accounts receivable is monitored on both a quarterly and an annual basis. By plotting all the information on one graph, the accounts receivable balance can be monitored graphically against industry benchmarks. In Figure 5.1, it is assumed that the benchmark accounts receivable balance is $4,000 per FTE veterinarian.

Graphing in this manner allows the numbers to be easily understood. In Figure 5.1 it is clear that accounts receivable is above the industry norm for the majority of the time. Both the days in accounts receivable and accounts receivable turnover ratios can be monitored in the same manner by comparing the practice's statistics with the industry median on a quarterly basis.

Benchmarking Productivity

Although it is beneficial to compare the productivity levels of veterinarians within the practice, it can even be more useful to compare them with those of veterinarians across the country. For example, productivity levels of veterinarians in a practice could all be very similar and considered acceptable, but when compared against national standards, they may, in fact, be very low, indicating certain changes are necessary. Productivity can be analyzed in a number of ways; the focus need not be only on revenue. Following are common productivity benchmarks that are used:

- Revenue per FTE veterinarian
- Visits per FTE veterinarian
- Compensation-to-revenue ratio per FTE veterinarian
- Hours worked per FTE veterinarian
- Average revenue per visit
- Average length of each visit

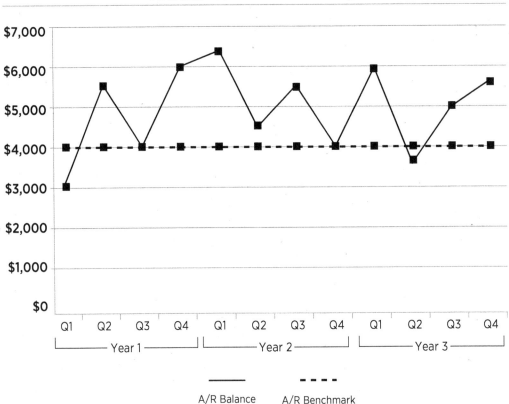

FIGURE 5.1
Accounts Receivable Benchmarking

Essentially, performing analyses for benchmarking is very similar to performing ratio analyses. Benchmarking simply takes the process one step further by comparing the productivity measures with external data to better understand the performance of the practice.

Benchmarking Expenses

Veterinary practices have many expenses, with the greatest usually being personnel. Although it is beneficial to benchmark a number of areas of a practice, it is often most useful to focus on the high-dollar areas. For example, benchmarking telephone costs (a small dollar item) will be much less useful than benchmarking personnel or drug costs.

With personnel costs consuming so much of the revenue generated, this is a very important area of focus. Personnel costs can be benchmarked for both dollars and number of staff. Basic benchmark comparisons include the following:

- Staff FTEs to FTE veterinarians
- Staff payroll and benefits or total personnel cost to revenue

- Personnel hours worked per patient visit
- Veterinarian compensation as a percentage of revenue and number of visits

Personnel costs tend to have the greatest number of benchmarks. Whether based on numbers of FTEs or on actual dollars, most benchmarking sources provide good comparisons for personnel performance. In most instances the staffing in a veterinary practice is not too volatile, meaning the number of FTEs and the salary levels do not fluctuate wildly on a weekly basis. Accordingly, it most likely makes sense to benchmark personnel costs on a monthly or quarterly basis to obtain useful information.

Also, when benchmarking personnel costs, it is important to separate veterinarian costs from general employee costs because most external sources will not include any veterinarian costs in their personnel benchmarks. This is a key example of how important it is to understand the benchmarking data and to ensure an "apples to apples" comparison is being made. In this situation, if the practice personnel costs included some veterinarian costs and the benchmarking source did not, the practice's personnel costs would appear to be extremely high, potentially leading the owner to take unnecessary action.

Other types of expense should also be compared against standards (e.g., medical supplies, drug costs, facility expense, marketing, and general and administrative costs). These can typically be compared as an actual dollar amount or a percentage of total revenue. Other expenses not usually part of overhead, such as interest, depreciation, and other noncash items, might also be separated from the ongoing operating expenses, but nonetheless are a central component of the overhead.

Sources of Benchmarking Data

Although there is limitless internal practice data for benchmarking, the external resources for benchmarking a veterinary practice are somewhat limited. Following is a list of resources available for veterinary practices to benchmark their performance:

- National Commission on Veterinary Economic Issues (www.ncvei.org), a Web site offering to its subscribers benchmarking and other assessment tools for evaluating and improving financial performance of the veterinary practice.
- American Animal Hospital Association (www.aaha.org), a professional organization providing accreditation, education, resources, and support for veterinary practice.
  - » *The Veterinary Fee Reference* (contains veterinary fee benchmarking data)
  - » *Compensation & Benefits* (contains compensation and benefits benchmarking data)
  - » *Financial & Productivity Pulsepoints* (contains revenue, expenses, and production benchmarking data)

- *Veterinary Economics* and other publications by Advanstar Communications (www .dvm360.com), which serves 60,000 veterinarians with financial information.
- American Veterinary Medical Association (www.avma.org), a professional organization that represents more than 78,000 veterinarians.
  - » *AVMA Report on Veterinary Compensation* (includes compensation and benefits benchmarking data)
  - » *AVMA Report on Practice Business Measures* (includes revenue, expenses, and production benchmarking data)
- *Veterinary Hospital Managers Association* (www.vhma.org), an organization that enhances and serves professionals in veterinary management through education, certification, and networking.
  - » *Practice Diagnostic Report* (personalized practice diagnostic report that provides useful and unique management statistics about your business)
  - » *Compensation and Benefits Survey* (includes compensation and benefits benchmarking data)

Although the external resources may be limited, this should not prevent a practice from engaging in the benchmarking process. These resources should be used to gather external data wherever possible. Also, the practice should network with colleagues and develop an information-sharing group wherein each practice could benchmark itself against the other practices in the group. This must be done in a legally compliant manner. VMG Groups, which are organized by an entity called Veterinary Study Groups, Inc.; Owen E. McCafferty, CPA, Inc.; and Professional Study Groups, Inc., allow veterinarians in similar practices to network and share best practices in a legally compliant manner. More information about VMG Groups is available at www.veterinarystudy groups.com. In addition, benchmarking can always be performed internally by comparing veterinarians within the practice as well as historical periods.

As mentioned previously, whatever the source of the benchmarks, it is essential to understand the data. Benchmarks should be accompanied by a thorough explanation of what the data are and how they were compiled.

It is important to monitor revenue, expenses, and other operational performance measures against benchmark standards. Although this requires more data collection, it is well worth it to compare a practice's operations with such definitive measures.

The use of benchmarking also helps to prevent a practice from thinking that it is different from all others and therefore does not need to change. This flawed thinking can be corrected by comparing industry standards with the practice's performance. The attitude that "we don't need to change" or "we have the right formula to fit our practice" can be influenced by the hard and comparative data that benchmarks provide.

Implementing changes in the practice can be difficult, especially in the face of politics and long-standing historical processes or perspectives. Reliable and comparable benchmark data, compiled over many years, can influence change and provide a credible mechanism for accountability.

Benchmarks are invaluable tools, important to the successful financial management of the practice. They can transform behavior when nothing else convinces those in the practice who resist change. Benchmarking is most effective when integrated into day-to-day operations. This is usually accomplished by processing the data, ensuring they are comparable, and then developing a well-organized system of management reports (including visuals such as graphs, charts, and tables) that translate the data into an understandable format.

SUMMARY

This chapter covers ratios and benchmarking, two important, even essential, tools for the successful financial management of the veterinary practice. Both should be used on a regular basis. Some may be useful on a daily or weekly basis, whereas others will provide relevant data only monthly or even quarterly.

Following are several prerequisites to ensuring success in calculating ratios and benchmarking the practice:

- The information should be compiled accurately.
- Outside information should be provided by reliable and proficient resources.
- The information should be used as a tool for learning and enabling change.
- The organization should be committed to using the data.
- Staff should be trained in how to use the information.
- Benchmark and ratio data should be presented succinctly.

Ratios and benchmarking may be the single greatest tool for implementing change that ultimately engenders success in the practice.

CHAPTER 6

Cash Management and Associated Internal Controls

In all business entities, cash is king. Without proper management and control of cash, operating a successful business can be extremely difficult. Facing competition, working with suppliers, and encountering outside forces are challenging in themselves. Practice owners must be wary of internal forces that may work against them and must be diligent in protecting the practice against loss.

Many businesses neglect to use their resources, such as banks and lenders, as assets. Instead, they view them as adversaries. This should not be the case. If cash is king, then practice owners should pay close attention to its uses and management. Basically, ensuring that proper control mechanisms are in place is a matter of instituting commonsense procedures. This chapter is about developing and accessing resources and implementing internal controls to ensure sound cash management and protection.

DEVELOPING BANKING RELATIONSHIPS
The Relationship Banker

In the not-so-distant past, emphasis was on the word *relationship* in banking relationships, and this is still the case in some instances. But many bankers seem more interested in selling products and generating short-term profits than in creating long-term relationships with their customers. Yet in smaller towns and communities where bankers have a vested interest in the community, small businesses may be able to develop better relationships with these banks than they can with larger banks and in metropolitan communities.

Regardless of locale and size of the community, the small-business owner's goal should be to cultivate a relationship with a banker, because this will pay off in the long term. When cash gets tight and a 30-day extension is needed on a loan, or if the practice is buying a new building or piece of equipment, it is good to have someone to call upon for both guidance and support.

The decline of the "relationship banker" is not entirely the fault of banks. On the one hand, in the competitive world of banking, it is easy for clients to move around to the institution that is offering the best deal of the day. On the other hand, the client who works with a specific banker and remains reasonably loyal can build a relationship that will pay off over the long term.

A banker should cultivate new businesses (by generating business loans and putting the bank's capital to work) and then receive those businesses' deposits from operating accounts (by putting this money into its coffers to lend to other businesses). Good bankers will offer advice and guidance—what interest rates are doing, how they view the overall health of businesses in the community, whether or not it is a good time to expand—not just make contact when they have a new product to sell or wait for customers to come to them. A good banker should be a good overall "business" person, someone who understands something about an individual's business, sales and marketing, the economy, and of course, banking. The banker should be available for clients to access his or her knowledge and understanding and should act as an advisor, an extension of the business that the owner would not otherwise be able to afford.

It may be difficult to understand for a new or small business, but there is significant value in having a relationship with a specific bank officer. It may be worth paying a bit more for a bank account or having an extra point on a loan. Consider the long term, and do not measure a banking relationship strictly by the fees.

Managing Bank Accounts

Most people have a bank account, perhaps more than one. So almost everyone has an idea how to manage an account: deposit money, write checks, use a debit card, or make withdrawals when necessary, ensuring the amount deposited will cover the amount taken out. Individuals have a checking account for paying their day-to-day bills and a savings account or money market account (MMA) where they keep money on a longer-term basis. This seems very straightforward, so it is perplexing that many people who operate small businesses tend to complicate their banking matters. This can occur for a variety of reasons, such as merging with another group that wants to keep separate accounts. Account management becomes very complicated when small business entities have multiple checking accounts for various functions. Managing multiple accounts is actually unnecessary.

There are advantages and disadvantages to using multiple cash accounts. On the one hand, employing minimal cash accounts, such as an operating account and a savings account or MMA, is most advantageous to a small business. Using one or two accounts is less costly and more efficient to manage. Using numerous accounts increases overhead expenses by requiring additional financial staff to manage them and by increasing the amount of bank fees.

On the other hand, using multiple accounts can offer many advantages to larger businesses, including separating certain funds from others, such as a subsidiary company or multiple subsidiary companies and their associated financial resources. Typically, larger organizations have a financial staff trained specifically to manage multiple cash accounts, with no additional staff or consequent expenses.

Usually, simplicity is more cost-effective in any business regardless of size, and this applies to having the smallest number of cash accounts needed to handle the business's financial resources. Although some advisors (e.g., accountants or financial managers) may recommend multiple accounts to segregate funds, this tends to turn an easy business into something more difficult to manage. A small business should have only one or two bank accounts, a checking account into which deposits are made and from which money is taken as needed, and another in which funds are kept for longer than 30 days and that might pay interest. More accounts will (1) cause more headaches, (2) require hiring someone to manage them, (3) cost more in fees, and (4) open the door for fraud. All segmentation of funds can be, and is best done, through properly establishing an accounting system (see Chapter 1).

Of course, the previous discussion refers to a single business entity. If an operating company, real estate company, leasing company, or holding company is involved, these bank accounts may have to be kept separate, primarily for tax reasons. It is good business not to commingle such funds, especially if there are multiple unique owners of the various other businesses and it is necessary to keep the money delineated.

Most banks not only want borrowers (a temporary activity); they also want to establish an overall banking relationship (ongoing business). Typically, establishing an overall banking relationship is in the best interests of a company, but it also benefits the bank itself. A company with operating accounts (or all of its accounts, for that matter) at a single bank may get better rates or more flexibility on loans or in other areas of the banking relationship, for a variety of reasons. First, the bank wants this business (i.e., the operating accounts) because it will usually charge a fee on the accounts. Also, if the bank has both the company's lending and its deposit business, the company will be more loyal and less likely to change banks. Finally, a strong banking relationship will often lead the owners of the company to bring their personal business to the same bank (i.e., personal account, home loan, etc.). An overall banking relationship also allows the bank to provide a better overall picture of the company's financial activity and feasibility.

A factor that may prevent a veterinary practice from keeping all of its deposits in one bank is the size of its accounts. The Federal Deposit Insurance Corporation (FDIC) insures loans with banks for each business only up to $250,000 (see posting at http://www.fdic.gov/deposit/Deposits/insured/basics.html), a fact that has become more important recently because of the failure of many banks as a result of losses in the sub-prime mortgage industry. This limit may not apply to all of the practice's accounts, depending on the practice structure, so it is important to ask the banker if the account is insured. As business volume grows and more money is added to accounts, it may be wise to consider opening additional accounts at other banks so that the practice's accounts do not grossly exceed the FDIC's deposit insurance guarantee. So there might be reason to diversify among banks.

When a relationship with a banker exists, the banker becomes a good resource. It is important not to jump from one bank to another just because the latter offers better terms on one product. Find a good banker who is in the know and understands the community. Consider this banker an ally, not a vendor who offers the lowest rates. There are many more important facets of a veterinary practice than regularly having to manage and be concerned about a banking relationship.

FRAUD AND EMBEZZLEMENT PREVENTION

Cash management challenges come not only from factors outside the practice (such as banking relationships; but also from internal factors. In addition to the risk that an unscrupulous employee will steal from the practice, there may be staff members who are hard-up and take money for purposes such as putting diapers on their children or food on the table. An employee may even decide that the owner makes too much money and that the wealth should be shared. The reasons given by embezzlers are numerous. Worse, those who steal look just like all the others; because they do not wear signs it may not be easy to distinguish the good from the bad.

To avoid the appearance of being overly suspicious of staff members and micro-managing the whole business, it is essential to have sound policies and procedures, avoid vulnerability, and use common sense. Once the money is in the door, some business owners assume it will get where it is supposed to go. Unfortunately this is not always the case.

Veterinary practices do not have as much to worry about as other health-care entities, in which much of the billing is done after the patient visit. Most practices receive payment at time of delivery via cash, check, or credit card, which substantially minimizes the management process, because there are no lengthy cash turnover cycles to incite worry. Regardless of the ease of payment or the method of payment, every practice should have a cash management process that ensures that (1) all required collections are made, (2) money is routed to the appropriate place, and (3) no fraud can occur.

The foundation for any cash management structure is twofold: (1) documentation and (2) process. These facets are discussed in Chapter 2, but that information is worth repeating here as it relates to proper cash management and fraud prevention.

Documentation

The two major components of documentation are the invoice and the receipt for payment. The invoice is the official statement of the services performed and the fees for the visit. Usually the veterinarian or technician completes the documentation at the time of the visit, which represents the start of the paper trail, or transaction tracking for automated practices. It is taken to the front-desk staff, who use it to determine how much to charge for the visit. When clients are checking out, they make the payment and then receive a receipt that documents what has been paid at that time. This is assuming that the client's balance for that date of service is paid in full. If it is not and the veterinarian wishes to extend credit and allow the client to set up a payment plan, this process will obviously not be as straightforward. If this is the case, there are now two pieces of paper, documenting how much was charged and how much paid, continuing with the paper trail. Without documentation there is no tracking; with no tracking there is no balancing; and if there is no balancing, then something is wrong with the numbers.

Process

The practice must have a straightforward billing and collections process to follow. In a veterinary practice this does not have to be unique to each and every occasion. Actually, the more efficient and streamlined the process, the easier it will be to follow. The discussion of the revenue cycle in Chapter 2 provides a good process to follow. Regardless of which system is adopted, it is essential to examine how cash is collected and the best mechanism to get it from the front desk/mailroom to the bank.

An important component of the process is the delineation of duties. This will include tasks like taking payment at the front desk, opening mail with checks in it, compiling deposit slips, and taking deposits to the bank. The goal is to structure the process so that duties do not back up to one another. This is like the "checkerboard" concept, where each point does not back up to or connect to another. This is more difficult in small organizations that have only two or three employees; the controls are much easier to establish in larger practices.

Preventing Fraud

The first purpose of managing cash flow (discussed at length in Chapter 2) is to make sure to get paid what is due for the services rendered. The second purpose of having a control system in place is to prevent occupational fraud and embezzlement in the practice. Systems designed for safeguarding assets are called "internal control" systems.[1] According to the *2008 Report to the Nation on Occupational Fraud & Abuse,* "occupational fraud" is "use of one's occupation for personal enrichment through the deliberate misuse or misapplication of the employing organization's resources or assets."[2] The report points out that health-care organizations are commonly victimized by fraud, with 8 percent of health-care organizations experiencing losses annually. Small businesses are especially vulnerable to occupational fraud. The median loss suffered by organizations with fewer than 100 employees was $200,000.[3]

In the most common scenario, a business owner ultimately discovers that a trusted, long-tenured manager has been swindling the company for ages. Theft is an age-old problem that is best dealt with by establishing safeguards that reduce the likelihood of it occurring. It makes sense to have the appropriate policies and procedures in place to prevent stealing. Policies and procedures are simple to administer. Following are suggested key policies and procedures to implement:

- **Separate duties.** Avoid using the same person to collect money from the front desk and to fill out the deposit slips and balance the money at the end of the day. If there are contiguous processes, break them up by inserting someone else to perform some of them. The employees may not like this because it takes longer or is less efficient, but this is an important separation of duties. Figures 6.1 and 6.2 are examples of good delineation of duties when dealing with cash paid at the front desk and checks received in the mail.

- **Rotate duties.** In small practices, everyone should be cross-trained whether there is an opportunity for fraud or not; this is good business and will provide needed support when a staff member is out. If someone is committing fraud and the practice is good about switching duties, discrepancies in the numbers should appear when staff members are doing different jobs.

- **Require mandatory vacations.** Although someone who works hard is a real asset, all those who touch the money should be required to take mandatory vacations.

They do not have to go anywhere—they can hang out at their homes if they want, but they simply may not come to the office and work during that period.

- **Look inward.** A business owner should compare numbers with benchmarks. Ideally, the practice's numbers should be higher, but even if they aren't, it should still use benchmarks to gauge where it stands. (See Chapter 5 for additional information about benchmarking.) If supply costs are running at 25 percent of revenue and benchmarks call for 20 percent, there must be a reason. Look for what is going into supply costs and make sure that a staff member is not paying for his or her groceries on the practice's tab.

FIGURE 6.1
Check Management Flow Sheet

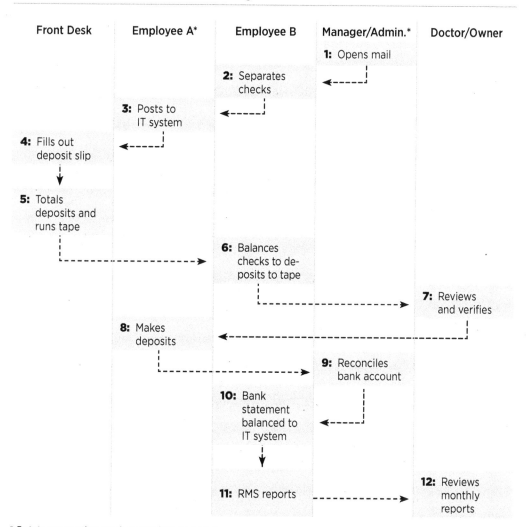

* Rotate every other week on random occasions.

FIGURE 6.2
Cash Management Flow Sheet

Front Desk	Employee A*	Employee B	Manager/Admin.*	Doctor/Owner
1: Receives cash				
2: Takes payment, writes receipt				
	3: Balances cash at end of day			
		4: Prepares deposit slip		
				5: Reviews deposit slip
			6: Makes deposit	

* Rotate every other week on random occasions.

- **Do spot checks.** Do different and unexpected things, although not to the point of being a nuisance to your staff and micromanaging everything they do. Take one day a month to sit down with front-desk personnel to balance the petty cash (see below). Or work with the person who puts together the deposit slip. You may never find any fraud, but you will learn how your business operates—always good to know.
- **Complete the basics.** Do things like balancing your financial statements, having an outside accounting review every year or two (at least), and reconciling your bank account routinely and consistently. These are all basic tasks every business should be doing, but many do not. Taking these actions will make it more difficult for others to perpetrate fraud against you; you will manage your financial statements better; and you will have a better idea of your financial position.

All of these preventive actions can be summed up in one phrase: Upset the apple cart. Get people out of their comfort zone and see how they react. See how your numbers change. Expect some resistance, as everyone is resistant to change, but it should be minor. Be wary of those who protest too much. If you see that things are different when one particular person is out—for example, money taken in per visit is a bit higher that week or expenses are a bit lower—this may not be the evidence you need, but it should prompt you to take the next step and look deeper. In addition, if employees know this is how you operate, then they will probably be less likely to take fraudulent actions in the first place. Instead, they will go work where there are less strict controls over the money!

What to Look For

Look for telltale signs that someone might have a tendency to commit fraud. You're not trying to identify a particular type of person, but rather looking for the things that embezzlers do to hide their tracks. Types of behavior you should watch for include the following:

- **Comes in early and leaves late.** Everyone wants a hard worker, the first to arrive and the last to leave, but unless you are grossly understaffed or are operating multiple business units, no organization consistently requires long hours of work. You should be wary of someone who is doing a lot of work when others are not there. Find out what that person is doing after hours that could not be done during business hours.

- **Is reluctant to release control.** If someone does not want to give up control and is unwilling to relinquish duties, you should wonder what that person is hiding.

- **Is disorganized.** Typically, people who are committing fraud will use covering behavior, such as being disorganized. If they are off $100 here or $200 there, they attribute it to their lack of organization, not to anything fraudulent.

- **Frequently makes mistakes.** This is similar to being disorganized, in that if someone is frequently making mistakes and entering incorrect data, it may not be because that person is incompetent; on the contrary, he or she may be very intelligent and trying to conceal fraud.

- **Constantly has computer system problems.** This is a big issue and is often very difficult to detect, because computer vendors never want to admit anything is wrong. If the person in charge says it is the computer company's problem, whom do you believe?

Minding the Small Money

In a small business, one would expect to notice if $100,000 were missing. So why would someone try to steal $100,000 from a business whose revenue may be only $1,000,000 per year? Missing 10 percent of the revenue would be pretty obvious! Someone who is intent on defrauding you will not go for the big bucks but will slowly milk the small dollars, $50, $100, $200 at a time. These amounts are difficult to track, and what's $50 in a $1,000,000 business?

Most embezzlers start small because they do not intend to start stealing in the first place. That is, they may need only $50 to make that week's rent, and they intend to pay it back; then the next week they need $100 to pay for another expense. Gradually the amount stolen grows, until it reaches $100,000, over the period of not one year but ten years! Fraud rarely ever starts as fraud, but rather as just an individual needing a bit more to make ends meet that month. Then it snowballs and the person is in too deep, as if suffering an addiction in which more and more is needed to feed the habit. People also become desensitized and rationalize their actions. The most common excuse is that the doctor/owner makes enough money, so what difference will $100 to $1,000 make? ("It's not like you *need* the money.") Finally, there is often a wide disparity between what a small-business owner makes and what the employees make. That is fine, but sometimes it causes owners to lose sight of lower-paid employees and not worry about a few hundred dollars. ("What can you do with an extra $100 a month?") Although the amount may not seem significant to the owner, some people live on razor-sharp margins, and to them it could mean a trip to the grocery store. Still, that does not make theft right. You must protect your business with controls and safeguards.

Prosecution

When you discover fraud in your practice and can prove that an employee has defrauded you and your business, you should prosecute. Embezzling money from you is little different from that same person walking up to you on the street and pulling a gun. Yet business owners seldom take the time to file legal charges, much less make the wrongdoer repay. The fact is that most people are repeat offenders, and if they were prosecuted and convicted, they would have a criminal record and could be prevented from doing this to someone else. Otherwise, they will continually put themselves in a position where they can embezzle from others. People with criminal records can be identified through background checks when they apply for employment. It makes good business sense to make fraudulent actions a permanent part of their history.

Unfortunately, for whatever reason, some victims of fraud do not press charges or try to recover the stolen money. It may be because of embarrassment, or that in the entire scheme of things it was not that much money. They may feel they would spend more money on an attorney than was stolen in the first place. However, if you don't seek retribution, you hurt yourself and likely that person's next employer.

CREDIT CARDS
Taking Credit Cards for Receivables

Every entity that benefits from cash at time of service (there are those that do not) should accept credit cards. Virtually everyone has at least one, and it is the most expeditious way to receive payment. You are paid at the time of service and the credit card company takes on any risk of nonpayment. Also, in cases when a client does not have the money to pay for a procedure, credit cards offer a way to finance these services, albeit a fairly expensive way (credit card interest rates range from 10 to more than 20 percent). In addition, the money is deposited directly into your account, so there is no cash exchange or checks that can bounce; credit cards are a very efficient way to manage your business.

Despite all of their benefits, credit cards have some drawbacks (i.e., fees), and depending on the card, these fees can be high. Do not think you are going to get all of the rewards without any cost! In some cases the fees are as low as 1 percent of the total charged, but for other cards, they can be as high as 5 percent. One card that businesses often do not accept because of high fees is American Express, but recently AE has become much more competitive, especially for small businesses. There are some pretty good deals available with AE for small-business owners, but you still need to keep these fees in mind. The other high-fee offender is airline and reward cards. Depending on the type of rewards, these fees are usually the highest, up to 5 percent.

Some small businesses simply do not accept cards with higher fees; others require the user to pay them. In the latter case the customer will usually just choose not to use that card. Some businesses are adamant about not taking certain cards because of their high fees, but they should consider what they are missing by not doing so. As in a banking relationship, credit card companies may provide access to a wealth of data they collect from their users, which can be very helpful the next time you plan a marketing campaign. Finally, as mentioned previously and discussed further below, with no exchange of cash, the opportunity for fraud and embezzlement decreases.

Using Credit Cards for Payables

The business owner must beware of fraud committed with employee credit cards. If a business needs a credit card, there should be only one card, not one for each person in the business. One person should control what goes on this card and what does not. If someone needs to buy something for the office (see also the petty cash discussion below), he or she should go to the person with the credit card and explain the need. If the card is used to buy supplies, the employee must keep receipts, and these receipts must be reviewed line by line by another person. Many business owners want to put everything they buy for their practice on a credit card to earn miles or other rewards. This is a good idea, but it allows small things to slip through the cracks. If you are charging $20,000 in supplies and equipment on your credit card each month, it will be difficult to notice the small $100 to $200 charges that should not be there. That said, if you do want to put all of your business expenses on a credit card, it should be a separate card with a separate invoice each month so that the other card can be checked.

Internal fraud using a credit card results from two activities: (1) charging relatively small amounts on the card for personal use, and (2) using an old card that everyone thinks is no longer valid. In the latter case, the user is still an employee and can intercept the statements before the owner sees them. Perhaps more egregiously, sometimes after an employee has been dismissed, he or she does not relinquish the credit card and continues to use it. In even more flagrant cases, some employees have actually applied for and received credit cards under the practice's name. In this case, it is wise to check your credit report for open accounts on a regular basis.

PETTY CASH

In today's era of credit and debit cards, there is little reason to keep petty cash on hand, especially when customers will be paying larger sums (more than $100). It is possible that cash will be used to pay for products that cost $20 or less, but this will probably be the exception rather than the rule. What is best for your particular practice should be discussed.

Petty cash is used for making change at the front desk and for buying small items for employees. Most payments at time of service should be made using credit/debit cards or checks. However, not all will be, so you may need to keep about $100 in the drawer. In most places it is, unfortunately, unsafe to keep a lot of money on hand, and customers should be made aware that it is safer for the practice not to accept large amounts of cash. As for buying small items for employees, it is much better to issue the office manager a credit card, as this can be used for nearly any size purchase. There is no need to have petty cash on hand for employee purchases, as credit cards are much easier to track and much safer to use.

When cash is used out of the cash drawer for change, the drawer should be balanced at the end of each day. Most modern cash registers will do this for you, and larger offices (especially ones that sell a lot of products) should use a register. In a small office, this may not be necessary. Nonetheless, you must balance the drawer at the end of each day. This is an easy, fast process, as outlined below, that is imperative to the safeguards discussed above:

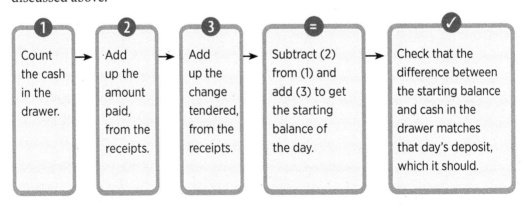

①	②	③	=	✓
Count the cash in the drawer.	Add up the amount paid, from the receipts.	Add up the change tendered, from the receipts.	Subtract (2) from (1) and add (3) to get the starting balance of the day.	Check that the difference between the starting balance and cash in the drawer matches that day's deposit, which it should.

Table 6.1 is a worksheet for following these steps. Daily balancing is a simple process that makes good business sense, though it is all too often overlooked. The only cash that should be kept on hand is a small amount for the change drawer; there is simply no need to keep business-related cash in the office.

TABLE 6.1
Petty Cash Reconciliation Worksheet

Starting Transaction No.	Total Balance	Amount Charged	Change Paid	Ending Paid	Balance
1	$100.00	$25.50	$40.00	$(14.50)	$125.50
2	$125.50	$15.00	$20.00	$(5.00)	$140.50
3	$140.50	$22.33	$25.00	$(2.67)	$162.83
4	$162.83	$55.00	$60.00	$(5.00)	$217.83
5	$217.83	$13.01	$20.00	$(6.99)	$230.84
6	$230.84	$22.00	$40.00	$(18.00)	$252.84
7	$252.84	$7.65	$10.00	$(2.35)	$260.49
8	$260.49	$14.99	$15.00	$(0.01)	$275.48
9	$275.48	$22.00	$25.00	$(3.00)	$297.48
10	$297.48	$19.25	$20.00	$(0.75)	$316.73
	$316.73	**$216.73**	**$(275.00)**	**$(58.27)**	**$316.73**

①		**②**		**③**		**=**		**✓**
$316.73 Cash in Drawer	→	**$(275.00)** Amount Paid	→	**$58.27** Change	→	**$100.00** Starting Balance ($(275.00) minus $316.73 plus $58.27)	→	**$216.73** Deposit

SUMMARY

There are many forces working against your veterinary practice that you cannot control. The market, the weather, your competition, and consumers may not all be trying to impair your success, but they often provide obstacles that you will have to overcome. Some people will want to harm you through fraud or embezzlement. This is why you must develop good relationships wherever you can and have strong internal controls and procedures to protect you when those who do want to harm you make it inside your operation.

Notes

1. Marsha Heinke, "Not in My Practice! Harsh Realities, Real Profit Potential," presentation to Ohio VBMA, October 22, 2008. Available at http://www.ohiostatevbma.org/webApps/vbma/assets/pdf/FraudEmbezzlementVeterinaryPractice. Accessed July 15, 2009.

2. Sidney Davidson et al., *Accounting: The Language of Business*, 7th ed. (Sun Lakes, AZ: Thomas Horton and Daughters, 1987).

3. *2008 Report to the Nation on Occupational Fraud & Abuse*. Available at http://www.acfe.com/documents/2008-rttn.pdf. Accessed July 15, 2009.

CHAPTER 7

Budgeting, Pro Formas, and Other Financial Planning Processes

The previous chapters discussed the evaluation of existing financial statements and assessing past performance. It is now time to look to the future.

Just as carpenters cannot build a house without a blueprint, an efficient financial planning process is essential for a veterinary practice to achieve long-term financial success. This chapter introduces a number of integral elements in the financial planning process: budgeting, pro formas, business plans, and feasibility studies. All are critical techniques for achieving long-term goals.

BUDGETING

Simply put, a budget is a money plan. Budgeting is a process of planning expense and revenue and measuring these values against the actual financial results. It can be considered a managerial tool that quantifies a practice's operational goals.

Budgeting functions can be performed by either outside accounting professionals or the practice management team. A variety of small-business accounting systems, such as QuickBooks™ and Quicken™, provide budgeting templates that help simplify the process.

Why Use a Budget?

Budgeting is widely used as a component of a practice's financial planning and expense control process. By evaluating the practice's specific economic condition and the near-term growth perspective, management sets up a reasonable budget, specifying the allowable expenses for future periods. These reasonable estimates (budgeting) then serve as operational goals and benchmarks against which performance can be evaluated.

From an operational management perspective, budgeting is essentially an action plan that allows management to monitor and control business operations in a quantitative manner. Periodic comparisons of budget versus actual performance provide management with indications of how the operational plans are being implemented.

The Budgeting Process
Who Should Be Involved?

Traditionally, budgets are created by the management team, including veterinarians, shareholders, practice administrators, and department heads. The budget may also be developed independently with the help of a designated financial professional. For smaller practices, managers may want to consult with independent accountants or consultants, who can use their industrial expertise to help develop a more sophisticated budgetary model.

For a budget plan to be carried out efficiently, it is advisable to allow as many staff members as possible to participate in the budgeting process. When staff members' job performance may be dependent on meeting the budget goals, budgeting can typically cause negative feelings among employees. Therefore, it is important for staff members to fully understand the budgeting process as a coordinated effort to achieve common objectives. This ensures that everyone is motivated to participate and comply.

Allowing staff to be involved in the budgeting process also creates a communication platform for members to share their hands-on input with the management team. This assists managers in refining the budget to reflect the practice's operational reality.

What Information Is Needed?

The best starting point for developing a financial planning process is always the historical data. Therefore, for budgeting purposes, the most important piece of information for establishing a realistic budget plan is the last three years' financial statements, in particular the income statement (also known as profit and loss statement). For practices that do not prepare an income statement, tax returns may be used.

The following information is also needed for the budgeting process:

- Last three years' productivity statements
- Lease documents
- Equipment lease documents
- Loan documents
- Fee schedule

- List of operational changes expected in the next few years and their consequent impact on revenue and expenses (e.g., new service lines, geographic expansion plans, changes in patient mix)
- List of major capital expenditures planned for the next few years
- Employee roster and most recent year's W-2s

For newly established practices that do not have historical track records, the planning process will rely largely on estimates. Under these circumstances, industry benchmark data and historical data relevant to similar entities would be useful.

Outside Influences on the Budgeting Process

The financial success of a veterinary practice is determined not only by how well it is managed internally, but also by the overall economic environment of the market it operates in. Because some veterinary services are considered consumer discretionary items, a number of outside factors must be taken into consideration when developing a budget for a veterinary practice:

- The **economic cycle** (also referred to as "business cycle"), which is predictable long-term pattern changes in national income. Traditional business cycles undergo four stages: expansion, prosperity, contraction, and recession. After a recessionary phase, the expansionary phase can start again. The phases of the business cycle are characterized by changing employment, industrial productivity, and interest rates. Some economists believe that stock price trends precede business cycle stages.[1] The economic cycle has an impact on consumer confidence, the labor market, and inflation, all of which affect a practice's ability to generate revenue. It is typical to see steady revenue growth when the economy is in the expansion phase and to see consumers cutting back on discretionary spending when the economy is contracting.
- **Technology.** New drugs or technological development often boost or reduce the demand for the services provided by a veterinary practice.
- **Interest rates and access to credit.** For entities that require outside financing, the level of interest rates and how easily they can obtain access to credit largely determine whether they are able to bring the potential investment or expansion projects to fruition.

Steps in Budgeting

Step 1: Determining the Desired Financial Results

Budgeting is essentially a financial planning process. To start this process, the practice must specify the goal it expects to achieve. This goal can typically be measured by profit, an absolute dollar amount that simply equals revenue less expenses. Or it can specify the earning percentage to revenue, a relative concept measuring the amount of profit that can be generated from each dollar of revenue received; this can be derived by dividing profit by revenue.

When setting goals for established practices, it is important to keep them realistic and attainable. This can be done by reviewing the practice's income statement for the past three years. How the practice has grown in the past provides a good indication of the amount of growth it can achieve in the future, assuming no dramatic operational changes occur. For start-up entities, the best way to set realistic goals is to utilize a lower percentile (for example, 25th) in the industry benchmark.

Keep in mind that goals must be refined and revised as circumstances change. For example, it is reasonable to expect profit to grow by 10 percent when the overall economy is in its expansion phase; however, a 10 percent profit increase may seem unrealistic if the economy exhibits a sharp downturn.

Step 2: Analysis of Financial Statements

Drawing up an effective budgeting plan requires a thorough understanding of the practice's financial resources. This is similar to knowing your income and where you spend most of your money when creating a personal budget.

The management team should perform an in-depth analysis of the most recent year's financial statement. This allows them to achieve a good understanding of the key elements of the business.

Revenue. Revenue is typically reported as a single line item on financial statements and tax returns. However, it is critical for managers to take time to understand the main sources from which the practice draws revenue, to identify key areas that possess the greatest growth potential. A common technique to better measure the historical trends and growth perspectives associated with each revenue element is to break down revenue by profit centers.

Depending on the operational structure of the practice, profit centers can be set up based on a variety of parameters, such as service lines (medical services, surgical services, laboratory services, radiology services, and pharmacy), veterinarians, and geographic locations.

A revenue breakdown report should be readily available from the cost accounting system for those practices that have such system in place. For those that have not established a cost accounting system, a good resource for obtaining revenue breakdown information is the productivity statements produced by practice management programs. If set up appropriately, practice management systems will allow users to sort revenue by veterinarians or billing codes, thereby providing revenue data at a much greater level of detail than do regular financial statements.

As discussed in previous chapters, there are a number of ways to assess a practice's ability to generate revenue, such as benchmarking and ratio analysis. These methods should be used whenever applicable.

Expenses. Normally a variety of expense items are reported on financial statements and tax returns. To simplify the analytical process and prepare for the budgeting process, expenses can be reorganized and compiled into four categories:

1. **Personnel Expenses:** Staff wages, payroll taxes, benefits, and other related expenses such as recruitment. Depending on the type of entity (e.g., sole proprietorship, partnership, or C corporation), owners' compensation may or may not be reflected on the financial statements.

2. **Occupancy/Facility Expenses:** Expenses related to the practice's facility, including rent, utilities, maintenance and repairs, and property taxes.

3. **Variable Expenses/Cost of Goods Sold:** Those costs closely related to the generation of revenue, which tend to change in direct response to volume, productivity, and/or revenue. Typical variable expenses are drug supplies and laboratory expenses.

4. **Fixed/Administrative Expenses:** The opposite of variable expenses; for the most part, they do not fluctuate with revenue changes. Although there is a relative range in which they may move, these expenses are not directly correlated with productivity; that is, these expenses will essentially exist no matter the patient volume. Examples of fixed expenses are business license and dues, advertising, equipment rental, and interest expenses.

Although it is relatively easy to identify personnel and occupancy costs, sometimes it is difficult to differentiate variable expenses from fixed expenses. A useful way of doing this is to run a correlation analysis (a kind of statistical calculation) between each nonpersonnel or occupancy expense item and revenue using a financial calculator or Microsoft Excel™. Variable costs typically exhibit high correlation (less than 85 percent) with revenue.

Once the expense reorganization is completed, routine analytical procedures (benchmarking, ratio analysis, etc.) should also be done on each expense category.

Step 3: Normalizing the Revenue and Expenses

Budgeting is typically completed by using the most recent year's income statement data. However, there may be extraordinary or nonrecurring items that will not continue into the future. This is especially true for practices that maintain financial records using cash-based accounting. When this is the case, management should consider removing these nonrecurring items or use the last three years' average to provide a normalized base-year figure to allow for more future projections.

Step 4: Budgeting Revenue

As discussed previously, projecting revenue on a per revenue/cost center basis allows for more accurate projections. These can be broken out by service lines, veterinarians, or geographical locations, depending on the specific situation of the practice. However, when that revenue breakdown information is not available, budgeting revenue based on the total figure is also acceptable.

Revenue budgeting and expense budgeting are closely related, in that the amount of revenue budgeted sometimes determines the level of expenditure required to produce that level of revenue. Relatively speaking, revenue budgeting is more difficult than expense budgeting because a number of factors must be taken into consideration. Some of these factors are discussed below.

Patient Volume. Patient volume is one of the key drivers of revenue growth. A number of external and internal forces can cause patient volume to change:
- Addition or discontinuation of service offering
- Addition or termination of veterinarian
- Veterinarians' ages and their ability and willingness to grow
- Changes in existing veterinarians' working hours
- Patient volume trend developed over the most recent three years and whether this trend is expected to continue
- Changes in geographical coverage
- Overall economic conditions and consumer spending trends
- Advertising and promotion activities
- Pricing changes
- Market competition
- Pet population growth perspective of the service area
- Demographic information associated with the service area, including population, age, gender, and household income

When developing patient volume projections, one must also keep in mind the constraints on a practice's capacity. An easy way to determine a practice's capacity is to look at its scheduling pattern. For example, assume a single-veterinarian practice sees patients every 15 minutes and procedures, on average, require one hour. Assuming two procedures a day, for every eight-hour working day, this practice can see a maximum of 24 patients (8 hours, less 2 hours for procedures, × 4 patients an hour). Based on 48 workweeks a year and 5 workdays a week, the practice's total capacity would be 48 × 5 × 24 = 5,760 patients a year. In other words, it would be unrealistic for management to project 8,000 patients a year for this particular practice.

Fee Schedule. Veterinary practices provide services mostly on a fee-for-service basis. Unlike medical practices, they rarely receive insurance payments. Therefore, a practice's revenue is driven by the way its fee schedule is set up and updated.

Fee schedule changes are easy to predict because they are determined by the management. However, it should be noted that merely increasing fee rates will not increase revenues commensurately. In most cases, higher fees will result in a higher risk of losing clients. This is especially true when a competing practice keeps its fees unchanged. For this reason, when projecting revenue based on an increased fee schedule, it is important always to consider adding a level of allowance for potential volume reduction.

Fee rates will be more difficult to budget if the practice is expected to realize additional revenue through the introduction of new service lines. For example, a practice's average fee rates may increase if new services that generate higher fees on a per unit basis are added. Use historical or comparable information when available. Otherwise, it may be necessary to conduct market research to determine a reasonable amount of fees that can be expected from the new service or to use pure speculation. In either case, estimates should be extra conservative.

After determining the future volume for each profit center and the corresponding fee rates, a revenue budget for each profit center can be calculated by multiplying the two elements. Total budgeted revenue will be derived by adding up the projected revenue for all the profit centers.

Step 5: Budgeting Expenses
Expense budgeting is relatively straightforward because, compared with patient volume, which tends to rely on overall economic conditions, expenses are more predictable as long as adequate information is available. Moreover, the four-expense-category structure compiled in step 2 provides a good platform to make expense projections easier.

As with revenue budgeting, the starting point of expense budgeting is the normalized figures from the previous year.

For expense projection, a simple method is to apply the last three years' average growth rates to the base-year figures. It should be noted that this method is applicable only to practices that meet the following three requirements:

1. The practice is established.
2. Expenditures were stable over the past three years.
3. The practice will continue operations in the future with a semblance of past operations.

For practices that do not meet these requirements, expenses should be projected on an individual basis through predictions about how future expenses will change in relation to the base-year figures. Typical expense budgeting procedures for the four distinct expense categories are discussed below.

Personnel Expenses. In most cases, staff wages comprise the majority of this category. Wage expenses can be estimated by applying an estimated raise percentage to the previous year's actual figure. For practices that may experience certain operational changes (e.g., adding service lines or veterinarians) during the upcoming year, management should also consider the potential adjustments in the staffing level as a result of such changes and project accordingly.

Payroll taxes and benefits usually change in direct proportion to changes in salaries. Therefore, a common way of budgeting payroll taxes and benefit expenses is to apply the historical average percentages as related to salary expenses to the estimated salaries.

In a small, privately owned practice (one or two veterinarians), the veterinarian-owner compensation is usually whatever is left over after all expenses are paid; this is easy to project. In larger entities, however, veterinarian compensation calculations usually entail complex compensation models that may even include a productivity incentive component. In these cases, management must review the actual veterinarian employment models thoroughly and project the compensation figures accordingly. It is important to project these expenses accurately because veterinarians' compensation is typically the largest expense in the practice.

Occupancy/Facility Expenses. Accurate occupancy expenses can be estimated by considering the terms specified in the leasing documents. Pay special attention to the escalator and additional rentals, as these are often overlooked when developing a projection.

Utilities and property taxes, if no additional office space is assumed, can be projected by applying an average percentage increase of the consumer price index (CPI) to the previous year's figure.

Variable Expenses/Cost of Goods Sold. Because these expenses are closely correlated with cost drivers such as revenue, productivity, and patient volume, they can easily be estimated by applying the particular expense's historical percentage of revenue.

Fixed/Administrative Expenses. For the most part, these expenses can be assumed to grow consistently with their average growth percentages for the last three years.

A few items may require individual projections. For example, equipment rental costs will be more accurately budgeted utilizing the actual rental payment schedule provided in the lease agreement. If the practice carries long-term, interest-bearing debt, the amortization schedules provided along with the loan documents will be helpful in determining the exact amount of interest expense in the next few years.

Step 6: Combining Budgeted Revenue and Expenses and Making Adjustments
Once the budgeting process has been completed for revenue and expenses, management can subtract budgeted expenses from the projected revenue figures to derive an estimate of future profits. This result is then compared with the desired profit determined in step 1.

When the budget indicates that more profit is needed than can be earned based on the revenue and expense budgeting, the following three types of adjustments may be considered:

1. **Increasing revenue.** It may be difficult to realize revenue increases because sales expansion cannot be realized instantly. Higher revenue may be obtained through increasing working hours, adjusting service offerings, or improving billing and collection functions (i.e., collecting as much as possible at the time of service). However, one must also consider the added expenditures associated with these changes.

2. **Lowering expenses.** Expenses can be adjusted relatively easily. To do so, management must differentiate the expenditures that are critical for the normal operation of the practice (e.g., rental, drugs, and personnel costs) from those that are discretionary (e.g., meals and entertainment, travel, gifts, fringe benefits). Expense saving can be realized by cutting back on discretionary spending and/ or choosing similar but less expensive items for nondiscretionary expenditures.

3. **Lowering targeted profits.** Under circumstances when budgeted profits are still below management's goal after expense and revenue budgets have been adjusted, the initially desired results may be unrealistic. It may be necessary to lower the profit target to a more attainable level.

Budget Control
Once the budget plan is set up, it should be carried out as a guideline for daily operational and financial activities. This can be done at practice, departmental, and individual levels.

Periodically, each responsible unit's actual performance should be appraised by comparing it against budgeted performance. Although slight variance may be accepted, a larger variance should be analyzed in depth. Variances can be caused by a number of factors, including noncompliance, waste, lack of sufficient control, and simply an unrealistic budget. Whenever variances occur, action plans should be made to resolve these issues.

Budgeting is a great internal control tool if implemented effectively. It can be used as a basis for rewarding or punishing. However, it should be used more as a tool for strategic alignment purposes to ensure that the practice's key profit contributor(s) are assigned sufficient resources for the entire practice to achieve its strategic goals.

Completing the Final Budget

Budgeting is an ongoing process. Entities will typically go through many revisions before a budget is finalized. An efficient budget plan will allow a practice to motivate employees, promote productivity, and ultimately boost long-term sustainable growth. The budget may also have to be altered to reflect changes in strategic development plans and other changes in circumstances.

PRO FORMA STATEMENTS

Pro forma is a Latin term meaning "as a matter of form." Pro forma statements are financial statements (including income statement, cash flow statement, and balance sheet) based on projections about the future.

Although public companies have long been required to disclose pro forma projections in compliance with Generally Accepted Accounting Principles (GAAP), it is optional for most small private firms such as veterinary practices. However, this does not mean that pro forma statements are meaningless for veterinary practices. Rather they are very powerful managerial tools to monitor financial performance and facilitate the decision-making process.

Pro forma statements could be used in a variety of scenarios. As discussed previously in this chapter, pro forma projections are an integral component of the budgeting process. Beyond that, financial professionals frequently develop pro forma analysis in support of a variety of business development initiatives, such as the following:

- Budgeting and monitoring
- Business start-up financing
- Financial and operational feasibility analysis
- Assessment of the cost-effectiveness of investment projects

Pro forma for veterinary practice budgeting purposes focuses on income statement items (i.e., revenue, expenses, and profits), but pro forma projections can also be developed for balance sheet and cash flow items. In fact, these are critical for estimates of financing needs for strategic development and financing purposes.

In most cases, pro forma revenue and expense projections can be prepared as a stand-alone report. However, the compilation of pro forma balance sheets typically requires pro forma cash flow and income statement projections to be completed in conjunction with each other. Given the interrelationship among the three pro forma statements, altering any one assumption in any of the pro forma statements will cause all three statements to change.

Although it is relatively easy to prepare a pro forma income statement, compiling pro forma balance sheets and cash flow statements will require solid accounting training. It is possible to engage an accounting professional to perform these services or use easy-to-use accounting computer software to complete these functions.

BUSINESS PLANS

A business plan is always one of the most important items on the checklist for starting a veterinary business. It is not only one of the documents lenders require as a part of the loan application package, but also an important exercise that allows veterinarians to formalize their ideas about the operations of the new business.

Pro forma projections are a key element of business plans. Unlike the budgeting process, pro forma places greater emphasis on cash flow projections. This is because one of the biggest problems for any business start-up, and also a major reason most ventures fail, is liquidity (the ability to generate sufficient cash to pay the bills and fulfill the interest and principal payments associated with debt obligations).

Similar to financial projections for all other purposes, start-up pro forma statements must be compiled based on realistic assumptions. Projections for start-up purposes are typically completed based on certain levels of speculation because of the lack of historical data. Therefore, it is better to be conservative in the construction of start-up pro formas and finance the project accordingly.

In addition to pro forma projections, business plans for financing purposes require a narrative description illustrating how the borrower intends to use the borrowed funds. This usually includes detailed action plans in the areas of marketing, market competition, operating procedures, and staffing. For new business ventures, it is also preferable to complete a demographic analysis of the intended service area.

Following is an outline of the basic elements of a business plan:

Operational overview
- Operational structure and management
- Mission statement
- Legal structure
- Administrative management

Marketing assessment

Business strategy

Financial management

Financial management structure

Accounting policies and procedures

Capitalization plan

Capital requirement

Capital contribution

Human resource requirement

Budgeting

Revenue source

Expense/overhead

Operating expenses

Veterinarian expense

Pro forma financial statements

Pro forma revenue projections

Pro forma expense projections

Personnel expenses

Occupancy expenses

Variable expenses

Fixed expenses

Veterinarian expenses

Pro forma income statements

Pro forma cash flow statements

Pro forma balance sheets

SWOT analysis

Strengths

Weaknesses

Opportunities

Threats

FEASIBILITY STUDIES

The feasibility study is a critical step in the business planning process. It provides a quantitative and qualitative measurement to help answer the question of whether a proposed project is financially viable. It differs from a business plan in that the latter is more concerned about how to turn a plan into reality. For this reason, feasibility studies are usually conducted before the business plan is developed.

Feasibility studies outline and evaluate several alternatives for achieving business goals and identify the most financially and operationally viable method given the assumptions and parameters set forth in the study process. It should be noted that feasibility studies do not provide assurance that the accepted project will in fact yield the projected returns.

Feasibility studies rely on pro forma financial projections, in particular the projection of future cash flows. In addition to profitability, feasibility analysis assesses each project's level of risk, which is reflected in the required rate of return associated with the project.

Along with a feasibility analysis, a sensitivity study is typically conducted by evaluating the effect of applying small changes to the assumptions under which the feasibility study is conducted. It provides a "what-if" scenario analysis that helps refine the feasibility study conclusions.

From a quantitative perspective, the conclusion of a feasibility study can typically be reached via a comparison of each alternative's net present value (NPV) and internal rate of return (IRR), two financial measures that reflect a project's estimated risk and profitability (cash flows). Again, these calculations require in-depth accounting and financial training, and a professional should be engaged to complete these tasks.

Feasibility studies should play an important role in helping practices determine whether they should venture into a new line of service, usually the acquisition of a rather expensive piece of equipment. Many practices will simply decide they want to pursue a venture without performing the proper level of financial due diligence. Thus, they will purchase the equipment and then realize that it is not a profitable venture, which can be the case for a variety of reasons. Prior to entering into new service lines, the practice should complete a feasibility study to determine if there is enough volume to support the new venture and if the revenue associated with the venture will exceed the costs. Depending on the results of the feasibility study, more analysis can be performed through developing pro forma financial statements relative to the new venture. This "homework" helps the practice enter into only those ventures that will add value to the practice in the long term.

CAPITAL ACQUISITION AND INVESTMENT SCENARIOS

Capitalization is usually acquired through debt financing or equity financing. Debt financing involves receiving funds from a bank, savings and loan association, credit union, mutual savings bank, finance company, insurance company, or specialty lender. For example, when a practice wants to purchase a new ultrasound machine, it may borrow the amount needed from its local bank. The agreement is memorialized in a loan agreement and comes with specific responsibilities. Conversely, equity financing is obtained from venture capitalists, veterinary groups, veterinary practices, or other health-care or investment entities. For example, a private investing group may wish to invest in a start-up practice that will specialize in some niche of veterinary medical care, often one involving advanced or emerging technology.

There are advantages and disadvantages to both forms of capital acquisition. An example is the divergent expectations for return on investment from each financing source. Debt lenders expect that the principal amount of a loan will be repaid in full, and they will be able to reap additional benefits in the form of the interest paid by the borrower. On the other hand, equity investors may or may not be guaranteed a return on their investment. Although the intention in a legitimate transaction is generally for investors to receive some form of remuneration for the use of their funds, this is not always possible. For instance, many start-up technology companies use equity financing. If the company is unable to create a marketable and financially viable product, the equity investor is at risk of losing the entire investment, without a chance for a return.

There are also differences in the supervisory capabilities and ownership stake attained when using debt and equity financing. Most debt investors, for example, do not become involved in the management or day-to-day operations of a practice when they provide a loan the practice will use to purchase an ultrasound machine. However, if a private investor provided the practice with a loan so it could purchase the machine, the investor may be granted oversight capabilities and a stake in the operation and management of the practice.

Most veterinary practices use both debt and equity financing to raise capital. However, this choice depends on the shareholders, owners, or partners in a practice; the practice's needs; and future goals. As an example, debt financing is typically used for the purchase of equipment (which is why a loan from a bank, rather than an investment from an equity financer, is normally used to purchase an ultrasound machine,).

One alternative to financing is leasing. There are two principal leasing arrangements: operating leases and capital leases. The primary difference between the two is that operating leases do not provide an opportunity for ownership, whereas capital leases generally do. This ownership may be conferred at the beginning of the lease or at fair market value at termination of the lease. It is important to note that leasing generally comes at a higher cost than traditional financing, even when ownership is not at stake.

SUMMARY

This chapter addresses using financial tools to plan for the future. Although some of the principles were introduced in previous chapters, the application here is for planning rather than management. The multiple applications of various financial statements highlight the importance of using these fundamental tools to attain operational stability and growth of the veterinary practice.

Note

1. http://www.investorwords.com/1641/economic_cycle.html.

CHAPTER 8

Supplemental
Financial Reports

The previous chapters of this book established a strong foundation for the overall financial management of a veterinary practice. This chapter builds on that foundation by
providing examples of useful financial reports for managing the veterinary practice.
The example reports presented here vary widely in presentation and appearance and
will likely vary widely from practice to practice. It is important that each practice use
the information contained in this book as well as the processes it already has in place to
establish its own reporting standards. The tools developed should be in direct response
to supporting these reporting standards and the priorities unique to each practice. This
chapter does not review the basic financial statements, as they were addressed in detail in previous chapters. Instead, it explores and provides examples of other reporting
mechanisms that can supplement the basic financial statements and provide useful information for the practice.

DASHBOARD REPORTS

Following is a list of "dashboard reports" that are used as warning signs to indicate
whether some form of action is necessary. Dashboard reports are analogous to driving
a vehicle or flying an airplane and looking at gauges to ascertain the performance levels
of important functions. These gauges tell the driver about a need for certain corrective
or other action. For example, if the fuel gauge shows empty, a predictable reaction occurs (i.e., finding a gas station and refueling the vehicle).

A well-run veterinary practice should have an efficient reporting system to gauge
performance. Those reports will be accurate, timely, succinct, and easy to read so that

the manager can draw conclusions and react appropriately. Thus, the capable manager of the practice will be equipped to make good decisions because of accurate and timely dashboard reports.

Just as a driver should look at the gauges in a car on a regular basis to make sure there are no signs of malfunction, dashboard reports must be reviewed regularly. With regular and consistent analysis, the manager and owner of the veterinary practice can easily monitor results, ascertain both positive and negative trends, and respond quickly. This is the essence of good financial management.

The following dashboard reports are broken down into three major categories:

1. **Productivity**
   Visits by veterinarian by site
   Revenue per visit by veterinarian by site
   Hours worked per veterinarian
   Revenue per visit
   Number of new patients per FTE veterinarian

2. **Financial**
   Income/expense statement components to budget and previous year by site
   Overhead as a percentage of revenue by site/department
   Collection percentage and bad debt
   Days in accounts receivable
   Accounts receivable percentage by aging category
   Credit balance summary report
   Staff costs (compensation and benefits) divided by revenue
   Staff hours worked
   Patient visits
   Veterinarian compensation as a percentage of revenue
   Average overhead cost per patient, excluding veterinarian salaries and benefits
   Departmental expense breakdown
   Key overhead categories (personnel, facility, variable, fixed) relative to revenue
   Marketing costs per new patient
   Revenue per FTE veterinarian

3. **Operations**
   Access wait time
   Wait time per visit
   Wait time for return call
   Collection agency collection rate
   Encounters worked per day

Number of appointment slots

Total appointment slots divided by total actual appointments

No-show rate

Number of new patients per FTE veterinarian

Staffing per FTE veterinarian

Patient cancellation rate

Number of referrals by source and/or veterinarian

This list is not comprehensive, as a dashboard report can be created for any piece of data that the owner and manager of the practice find useful in terms of managing the practice. Most of these are self-explanatory and can be generated from good practice management and accounting systems. If these systems are not currently formulated to generate certain reports, most often they can be created through customization of the reporting tool. In many instances, the data are available; it is just a matter of choosing the proper report to generate the information needed. Some information systems may be able to export data into a spreadsheet such as MS Excel™, Lotus Notes™, or MS Access™. This allows for further customization of the data and reporting process to modify them into a more useful format.

Some of the aforementioned reports have been discussed and illustrated throughout the book; several are also illustrated throughout the remainder of this chapter. The intent is to explore their specific use as supplemental financial management tools.

FLASH REPORTS

"Flash reports" illustrate basic summary data for the entire practice. They are overall summaries of practice performance that may be completed at regular, defined intervals (at least monthly) and presented for management review. These reports are typically compiled by the financial manager of the practice and distributed to each veterinarian. In some instances, the sharing of financial data is limited to the owners, but other practices share the data with all veterinarians. Each veterinarian can use the report to draw his or her own conclusions, or it can serve as a basis for discussion in regularly held management meetings.

The key to using flash reports is that the layout and the data provided should be basic and easy to digest, but very informative about the day-to-day operations of the practice. Key data should be included, such as revenue, overhead expense, number of patients, and number of new patients. This information should be easily comprehended by all users, regardless of their financial and operational knowledge. Table 8.1 is an example of data that should be digested each period.

TABLE 8.1
Flash Report Reflecting Key Financial Metrics

| | CURRENT PERIOD | | YEAR-TO-DATE | |
	Year 1	Year 2	Year 1	Year 2
Sales—Service	$150,000	$142,000	$600,000	$568,000
Sales—Retail	$12,000	$12,500	$48,000	$50,000
Overhead	$75,000	$72,000	$90,000	$33,000
Patients	1,000	940	4,000	3,760

Expenses as a Percentage of Net Revenue

Staff Compensation	22.00%
Benefits	6.00%
Drugs	20.00%
Administrative	7.00%
Facility	13.00%

Another type of flash report may compare performance data with a budgeted figure or goal the practice has established. Table 8.2 is an example. Alternatively, benchmarking data may be loaded into the report to assess the financial and operational performance of the practice next to its peers. This type of report can quickly provide data on the financial performance by illustrating trends from prior periods or compared with other data sets.

TABLE 8.2
Flash Report Comparing Performance Data with Budgeted Figures or Established Goals

	Goal	Current Month	Previous Month	YTD (2 Months)
Revenues	$50,000	$45,000	$48,000	$93,000
Overhead (total)	$41,500	$39,000	$42,000	$81,000
New Patients	46	50	40	90
Total Patients	180	165	175	340
Expense Ratio	83.00%	86.67%	87.50%	87.10%
Profit (loss) (cash basis)	$8,500	$6,000	$6,000	$12,000
Net Income Percentage	17.00%	13.33%	12.50%	12.90%

DETAILED REPORTS

The following sections illustrate various management reports that can be used for financial analysis in addition to the basic financial statements. These differ from dashboard reports in that they provide much more detailed information and likely will be used less frequently. Most likely, these types of reports would be compiled quarterly, but on occasion monthly.

Productivity Reports

One basic yet very telling productivity report is increase in patients over a period of time. Table 8.3 illustrates practice productivity trends distinguished by new and established patients. This report may be made even more detailed by separating by veterinarian, or can be looked at on a more "micro" basis by separating by quarter or month.

TABLE 8.3
Increase in Patients over a Five-Year Period: New and Established Patients

	Year 1	Year 2	Year 3	Year 4	Year 5
New Patients	431	467	513	522	607
Established Patients	4,210	4,599	4,943	5,456	5,874
Total	**4,641**	**5,066**	**5,456**	**5,978**	**6,481**

Once the data have been gathered, inferences can be made about the growth trends. For example, in Table 8.3 the total patient growth was approximately 8.4 percent from year 4 to year 5. The growth in new patients was approximately 16.2 percent, whereas the growth in established patients was lower.

An example of a more detailed productivity report is Table 8.4, which examines the various veterinarians, days worked per veterinarian, and visits per veterinarian and determines the average visits per day. This report offers much insight into each veterinarian's true productivity. Although one veterinarian might have more cumulative patient visits, if he or she works a greater number of days, the average patients seen per day may be much lower than for his or her peers, or even lower than acceptable benchmarks. This report attempts to peel back the layers to get to the actual picture of performance.

TABLE 8.4
Detailed Productivity Report: Patient Visits

Because the high variability among practices would affect the data being presented, data are not included in this table. Please fill in representative data for your practice.

Provider	Days Worked	VISITS		VISITS PER DAY	
		Office	Total	Office	Total
A	_____	_____	_____	_____	_____
B	_____	_____	_____	_____	_____
C	_____	_____	_____	_____	_____
D	_____	_____	_____	_____	_____
Total	_____	_____	_____	_____	_____

Another type of productivity report that might be used on a regular basis considers veterinarian productivity distinguished by type of service. Table 8.5 is an example of such a report. It breaks down productivity by office visit, procedure, and radiology (i.e., x-ray and other imaging modalities), but other categories may be added that fit the service offerings of a particular practice.

These detailed productivity reports can also be expressed in the form of actual dollars or even percentages. This widens the array of data reviewed and available, which further increases the ability of the practice to make strong financial and operational decisions.

TABLE 8.5
Detailed Provider Productivity: Type of Service

Because the high variability among practices would affect the data being presented, data are not included in this table. Please fill in representative data for your practice.

Provider	Office Visit	Procedure	Radiology	Total
A	_____	_____	_____	_____
B	_____	_____	_____	_____
C	_____	_____	_____	_____
D	_____	_____	_____	_____
Total	_____	_____	_____	_____

Revenue Reports

On an overall basis, the practice can illustrate its revenue and other key data pertaining to the generation of fees. Table 8.6, which illustrates comparative revenue, visits, and revenue per visit, is for a period of five years. Of course this type of report can also be broken down by veterinarian or into smaller periods of time, such as months and quarters. The table is concise and easily understandable, thus making it an effective decision-making tool. Of course, as more detailed data are added, such as per veterinarian data, or for shorter periods of time, the report will become more difficult to analyze and use to draw appropriate conclusions.

TABLE 8.6
Comparative Revenue, Visits, and Revenue per Visit

Period	Visits	Revenue	Revenue/Visit
Year 1	9,000	$1,100,000	$122.22
Year 2	10,000	$1,200,000	$120.00
Year 3	11,750	$1,600,000	$136.17
Year 4	11,500	$1,650,000	$143.48
Year 5	12,000	$1,800,000	$150.00

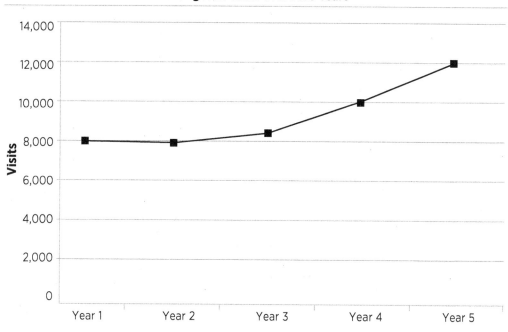

FIGURE 8.1
Changes in Visits over Five Years

Such tables can also be illustrated graphically; this often allows conclusions to be drawn more readily. This is because wild swings in the data or inconsistent trends tend to show up to a greater extent in a graph than in a list of numbers. When using spreadsheets such as MS Excel™, graphs can easily be created by the click of several buttons. Figure 8.1 is a very simple example of such a graph. It illustrates the changes in visits over five years. Another alternative is to plot both visits and revenue, and then compare trends between the two different measures of productivity.

Expense Analysis

The consideration of revenue is an essential part of the financial review process, but expenses should not be overlooked. Often the proper control and oversight of expenses can have just as great an impact on the bottom line as increases in revenue. Accordingly, expenses should always be considered a key component of the financial review process. It is beneficial to perform high-level calculations on expenses in total, but they should be broken down in greater detail as well. The key is to look at as much detail as possible without it being overly cumbersome. When too much information is presented, it often becomes more difficult to analyze, resulting in fewer conclusions to be drawn. Thus, a proper balance must be established. Typically this can be done by grouping expenses into meaningful categories, such as the following:

- Personnel costs
- Facility costs
- Variable costs (cost of goods sold)
- Fixed costs (administrative)
- Veterinarian costs

For a veterinary practice, analyzing expenses in these five main categories should provide an appropriate level of detail. If there are questions about a particular expense category, additional detail can be obtained to further analyze the variances.

The practice manager and owner should look at expenses in a number of different ways, such as the following:

- Common-sized (as a percentage of revenue)
- Total expenses by veterinarian
- Average overhead per patient
- Expenses per service line (i.e., ancillaries, etc.)

These expenses should also be compared against prior periods as well as the established budget. This will allow for trends to appear that allow the practice to better assess its performance. It is difficult to draw conclusions from only a single period of expenses, and comparing month-to-month or a quarter's worth of activity with the budget for that quarter allows for a more thorough analysis. Examples of supplemental expense reports are discussed below.

Table 8.7 is an example of a tool for analyzing the overhead costs on a per patient basis. These data normalize the level of overhead based on the number of patients, so that the practice can better understand how its overhead is trending in relation to the number of patients seen.

TABLE 8.7
Report Analyzing Overhead Costs on a per Patient Basis

Because the high variability among practices would affect the data being presented, data are not included in this table. Please fill in representative data for your practice.

	OVERHEAD (excluding provider costs)	OVERHEAD Patients	Per Patient
Example:	*$225,000*	*3,000*	*$75.00*
Q4, Year 1			
Q1, Year 2			
Q2, Year 2			
Q3, Year 2			
Q4, Year 2			

TABLE 8.8
Common-Sized Expense Analysis

	Year 1	Year 2	Year 3
Revenue	100.00%	100.00%	100.00%
Personnel	27.00%	29.00%	25.00%
Facility	6.00%	6.50%	6.25%
Variable	24.00%	23.00%	27.00%
Fixed	14.00%	13.00%	14.50%
Provider	29.00%	28.50%	27.25%

Table 8.8 is an illustration of this information. Of course, this type of analysis may be much more detailed; the example merely illustrates the concept. The report actually used by a practice should be modified to include the metrics that are most pertinent to its operations.

The practice should create several key expense reports to be distributed to the practice manager and owner and reviewed on a regular basis.

Individual Veterinarian Analysis

In addition to reviewing reporting data on revenue and expenses (mainly overhead), it is important to take a regular look at the trends occurring in veterinarian compensation. The intent of these reports is to ensure that all veterinarians are being compensated fairly in relation to the work they are performing. This is especially necessary in a practice with multiple owners.

Table 8.9 is an example of a report that can be used to calculate ratios of compensation to collections and visits, and allows a user to draw inferences about the appropriateness of compensation for the respective levels of productivity. Assuming an equal ownership scenario, if all veterinarians are producing at nearly the same rate, it would be reasonable to assume that their compensation should also be similar. Compensation should likely vary for differences in productivity; a higher producer would receive a higher level of compensation than a lower producer. However, when calculated as a percentage of production, their compensation should be similar.

TABLE 8.9
Report for Analyzing Veterinarian Compensation

	Revenue	Visits	Compensation	Compensation/ Revenue	Visit
Provider A	$486,000	3,600	$121,500	25.00%	$33.75
Provider B	$612,000	3,840	$146,880	24.00%	$47.81
Provider C	$396,000	2,880	$87,120	22.00%	$30.25
Provider D	$306,000	1,680	$64,260	21.00%	$26.78

SUMMARY

Summary schedules are an essential part of the financial reporting process. The typical financial statements (i.e., income statement, balance sheet, statement of cash flow) are important and necessary; however, more detailed summaries facilitate a more thorough financial analysis and decision-making process. Each practice should review its financial data needs and formulate reports that provide the data that fulfill these needs. This chapter illustrates the types and functions of some of these reports.

The flash reports discussed above are most informative when utilized on a frequent basis. At the very least, these reports should be reviewed monthly, but better weekly or even daily. The dashboard reports are more useful on a monthly basis, as it will be more difficult to draw inferences and conclusions regarding the data when they are presented more frequently. Finally, the more detailed reports should be reviewed less frequently, such as quarterly or annually. Of course, if a practice finds them useful, they can be utilized more frequently.

A successful veterinary practice depends largely on the ability to capture, report, and review meaningful financial data. Accordingly, an information system that provides accurate and quality data is necessary in every practice. Of course, this is only the first step. The practice must also have individuals who can extract the data from the system and review the information, drawing conclusions that can lead to better management of the practice. Furthermore, these individuals must be able to implement changes based on the conclusions drawn and continuously monitor results for additional changes that may be needed.

CHAPTER 9

Information Technology and Financial Management

Only between 5 and 10 percent of veterinary practices nationwide use completely paperless, electronic medical records (EMR) systems. However, veterinary medicine, like human medicine, is evolving in many strategic areas, particularly medical records management. Moving to an EMR system is perhaps one of the easiest and most efficient ways to increase productivity and reduce operating costs. There is currently a strong push to move into a paperless environment because of the efficiency and savings associated with the utilization of EMRs. This chapter reviews the vital role that information technology (IT) plays in practice operations and financial performance for the veterinary practice and guides the purchaser in making sound technology decisions.

GOING PAPERLESS

For the veterinary practice, there are many quantifiable advantages to moving from paper records to an EMR system:

1. **Improved efficiency.** An EMR system can make daily tasks, such as capturing patient visit data (SOAP), documenting progress notes, creating surgical records, updating problem lists using standardized diagnostic codes (for example, the AAHA Diagnostic Terms), renewing prescriptions, and reviewing lab results, much faster and easier. It allows users to view all applicable patient information in one place. Paper charts are notoriously difficult to keep track of and must be constantly retrieved from and returned to storage. The design of paper charts allows for a very limited amount of organization. An EMR allows instant access to essential information needed to complete a patient visit.

2. **Space saving.** Eliminating file cabinets, folders, and storage boxes means less room dedicated to records and record keeping and possibly more room for patient care.

3. **Cost savings.** Less administrative work is required when there are no records to file or retrieve each time an appointment is scheduled or a client calls. Staff members simply pull up records on a computer to access client or patient information and electronically record desired information.

4. **Improved staff morale.** Veterinary staff enjoy the benefit of spending more time in patient care and client interaction, instead of filing or retrieving patient records. Many staff members (especial ly younger veterinarians and staff) are extremely comfortable with technology and view skills in using it as necessary for success.

5. **Improved practice image and marketing efforts.** Clients tend to perceive practices with electronic systems as more progressive or up-to-date, and thus the veterinarian and staff as more knowledgeable. Features such as e-mail and a practice Web site with automated features and useful information for clients are especially appealing.

6. **Reduction of user error.** Prompts or pop-ups flag patients' allergies, drug interactions, as well as special considerations, account balances, and other items for clients. Protocols can be designed and implemented to tailor the program to the practice.

7. **Automated functionality.** In-house lab data as well as some outside laboratory results can automatically transfer into patient records. Radiographs, ultrasound images, electronic monitoring results, and other digital images can also be captured. Prescription instructions can be made in advance and automatically linked to certain procedures or billing items, and then be personalized before they are given to the client. Invoicing charges can be generated by the medical record entries, eliminating the potential for many charges to be missed.

8. **Ease of use.** Thanks to improved user interfaces, software programs are easier to learn for people with or without prior computer experience, and minimal typing ability is required.

Many factors are involved in selecting a computer system, and comparing vendors and products can be daunting. Several companies offer solutions for veterinary practices, each claiming to be the best. When a practice is contemplating opening a new office or adding new technology, a computer system will be essential and one of the more important decisions. The ability to manage medical records and finances electronically is a must in today's high-tech world. So where does the decision process begin?

New systems today are much more complex than in the past, going beyond just basic accounting software. Most vendors today offer fully integrated systems that include accounting, inventory management, retail medications and purchasing solutions, and EMR systems built on a single platform. Because of this, the decision to purchase a system is now much more critical and long-lasting. The economic ramifications of a poor decision are also much greater because the system will affect all components of the medical practice.

Choosing Software

All experts will advise that it is important for a practice first to understand and define its own needs. Too often, a practice jumps into the decision to buy a computer system without defining its expectations and key vendor requirements. It is important not to assume that buying a new system will solve all practice problems. Most new owners are on a limited budget and need to know the system will perform as expected and that the vendor will meet their expectations. Therefore, begin with outlining the needs of the practice.

Define Practice Requirements

Each practice has unique requirements that must be understood and documented. Vendors will do a much better job demonstrating their software's capabilities if given specific expectations in advance. The process of defining needs will require an objective evaluation of current processes. This can be very difficult for some practices because it requires admitting that certain processes are flawed or that change is necessary. Going from paper to electronic can be uncomfortable for those who are not familiar with computers. Following is a checklist for gathering information about a practice that is needed to define needs and objectives:

1. **Establishing a small work group.** This should consist of members from each department in the practice. The work group will encourage group participation and provide a broad range of viewpoints.

2. **Examining current workflow.** Have the members of the work group review their own departments and encourage all employees to contribute information about workflow and operations. This will serve two critical objectives. The first is to develop a global understanding of current processes. The second, and most important, is to flush out any operational threats or points of failure.

   a. How is scheduling handled?

   b. Are there other resources that should be scheduled (i.e., procedure room, surgeries, kennel availability)?

   c. How are walk-ins handled?

    d. What information is gathered and collected at the time of registration?

    e. How are appointments confirmed?

    f. Are scheduling reports needed?

3. **Technical assessment.** To know what the practice needs requires first knowing what it has. Technical assessments should be completed by someone who is qualified and knowledgeable in computers, security, and networking. The following items should be inspected:

    a. Equipment locations, including servers, workstations, and networking equipment:

        i. The servers should be located in a low-traffic area.

        ii. The servers should be located in an area that has environmental controls 24 hours a day, seven days a week.

        iii. Dimensions of equipment—current and future.

        iv. Space required to support the equipment.

        v. Is the space accessible, and is there room to work?

        vi. Workstations must be accessible in each exam room as well as in other areas throughout the practice where access to medical records is needed.

        vii. What types of workstations are preferred: stand-alone, dumb terminal, tablet PC, notebook, netbook, PDA?

    b. Electrical requirements:

        i. A dedicated outlet should be available for each server. Failure to supply this type of outlet could result in voiding the warranty with the server manufacturer. Install the type of outlet indicated, not more than four feet from each server's location.

        ii. All peripheral devices should have 110-volt outlets. A surge protector is recommended for all computer/printer equipment. Two receptacles are required for all workstation locations and network printers that do not have a built-in network interface.

    c. Phone lines and Internet connectivity:

        i. What is the current bandwidth?

        ii. Who will support and set up connectivity?

        iii. Is there adequate space to install networking equipment?

    d. Cabling requirements:

        i. Minimum CAT 5 cabling should be provided, with each end labeled properly.

        ii. Will the switch/hub and patch panel support all the additional computers?

    e. Existing equipment and software.

    f. Data conversions (only if an existing system is already in place).

    g. Develop an infrastructure diagram of both the network and hardware.

4. **Assessment of staff and their ability to adapt to change.** The greatest obstacle to implementation of EMR is the people factor. Building into this assessment the looming factor of aversion to change and how to deal with it helps a practice prepare for bumps in the road.

5. **Scheduling.** This is a major factor in workflow and should be well understood and documented. The scheduling process sets all other activities in motion and triggers several events. Knowing what works well and what does not will help in selecting a system best suited for the practice.

6. **Registration.** This function should also be included in the assessment for an integrated financial/EMR system. The following areas should be analyzed:
   a. What is needed for new patient registration?
   b. How are demographic updates handled?
   c. How does the practice management (PM) system assign account numbers that are needed for interfacing?
   d. Are travel sheets/super bills and invoices up-to-date, or will changes be necessary?

7. **Current methods for manually capturing medical records.** Examining the current methods will produce a lot of helpful information about processes that need conversion over to an electronic record-keeping system.

8. **Phone calls.** Documenting calls will require extensive revamping with EMR. Knowing how processes are handled today will allow the practice to select a vendor based on its ability to make the most significant improvements. The practice should also consider how after-hours calls and remote access are handled.

9. **Medical records (SOAP, notes, surgeries, etc.), prescriptions, labs, and orders.** These are all significant components of the workflow that will be affected by EMR. Consider these areas:
   a. Who is responsible for creating and completing medical records (outpatient and hospital cases), importing laboratory data, capturing and linking digital images, and handling prescription refills, and how is the process communicated? Who has access to various parts of the medical records? How are medical record entries documented, including name of entry user, date, and time? How are changes to medical record entries tracked?
   b. What are the policies for
      i. calling in prescriptions?
      ii. dispensing in-house medicines, both prescription and over-the-counter?
      iii. dispensing samples?
   c. How is educational material for the client handled?
   d. How are treatment, lab, and radiology orders handled?

    e. How are lab and radiology results handled?

    f. How are lab and radiology results reviewed and documented?

    g. How are lab and radiology results communicated to clients?

Contact Vendors

After defining requirements, the next steps will be to contact vendors and request a product demonstration. A demonstration can be done over the Internet, but it is better to have the vendor do the demonstration in person and allow for some hands-on interaction. Consider the following demonstration tips:

- Limit demos to three or four hours. Time constraints help vendors stay focused.
- Selected team members should include a cross section of users. Have the same team members evaluate all demos.
- Do not allow vendor representatives to outnumber selection team members.
- Ask vendors to use a projector so everyone can see.
- Save the demos for your final two to five vendors—preferably only two or three.
- Inform vendors they will be evaluated based on objectives defined by the practice.
- Do not allow a demo of a product that is not yet ready. Do not accept vaporware (i.e., products that are yet to be developed or are still being tested)!
- Do not make the demo the sole determinant of the selection decision.
- Make vendors show rather than describe. Do not allow a vendor to just say that something works; insist on seeing it!
- Is the version being demonstrated the same as what will be purchased?
- Listen for contradictions.
- Ask lots of questions. The more questions asked, the more likely it is that contradictions will arise.
- Leave time for hands-on demonstration.
- After the demo is finished, dismiss the vendor and ask the selection committee/work group to remain in the room.

After demonstrations are finished, there should be a preferred vendor. The next major step is to ask for a list of customers and complete reference checks, keeping in mind the following:

- Issues to discuss with the vendor's other customers include the following:
  - » Why that customer selected the software
  - » System performance versus expectations
  - » Quality of training provided
  - » Performance of implementation team
  - » Ability of vendor to meet schedules and deadlines

- » Attitude of vendor staff (friendly, adversarial, etc.)
- » Problems during implementation and how they were resolved
- » How bugs were handled
- » How new releases/upgrades were handled
- » Unexpected surprises (good and bad)
- » Challenge of finding and retaining IT talent to support the system
- » Major benefits of the system
- » Major limitations of the system
- » Vendor responsiveness to support and maintenance problems
- » What the hidden costs were
- » Whether or not there were customization issues
- » How the vendor handled difficulties
- » Whether or not the vendor tried to blame others or took responsibility
- Open-ended questions should be used.
- And finally, ask, "If you had it to do all over again, would you still choose the same vendor?"

In many cases a customer who has complained about the vendor throughout the reference call will still choose the current vendor. It is best to talk to several references to see if there is an emerging trend. If most of the references are positive, then chances are good the vendor will live up to expectations. If most are negative, there would be reason to be concerned and possibly avoid this vendor.

Examine Clinical Content

When selecting an EMR, it is important to inspect the system for clinical terms specific to the treatment of animals. Make sure that the system has clinical content such as diagnostic terms, commonly prescribed medications, and treatment plans. This will result in spending less time and expense to incorporate these terms into the system manually after the purchase. AAHA offers commonly used diagnostic terms that should be embedded in the EMR.

Negotiate with Vendor

The last task is to negotiate a contract and the terms and conditions of the financial arrangement for procurement of the new system. Successfully negotiating a vendor contract is the final act in a thorough selection and planning process. To ensure a successful negotiation, follow these steps:

1. Identify vendor costs for *all* functions: fixed, ongoing, present, and future. Here are a few areas to look for:

    a. Initial costs

    b. Hardware cost

    c. Software cost

    d. Communications cost

    e. Installation cost

    f. Implementation cost

    g. Ongoing support cost

    h. Integration costs

    i. Interface cost

    j. Entitlement to new releases/bug fixes

    k. The cost of tailoring

    l. Future upgrades and releases (these should always be at no additional cost)

2. Recognize various software features and how they affect costs. For example, a Web portal may be supplied by a third-party vendor that will also expect payment. Vendors will frequently use third-party databases for live art, dictionaries, and formularies. These databases typically require an annual renewal fee.

3. Address software customizations, especially integration requirements.

4. Gather competitive data, and always have a viable second choice. Let both vendors know they are under consideration.

5. Develop a quote comparison spreadsheet or chart (see Figure 9.1).

Negotiating successfully is getting to the rock-bottom price, with the vendor doing the digging.

Review the Proposed Contract and Negotiate the Terms and Conditions

The contract review process should include both a business and a legal review. Some organizations specialize in vendor contracting and procurement and can offer assistance in reviewing these types of contracts. A legal review by qualified counsel is also advisable.

To prepare for contract negotiations, develop a list of all issues to be negotiated. Define the issues and the desired outcome. Prioritize the list and identify nonnegotiable criteria. Sort the items into deal-breakers, neutral, and "wish list."

Following are key points to include in your contract review:

- Implementation plan
- Software customizations
- Criteria for acceptance
- Terms of payment
- Software and hardware maintenance fees

FIGURE 9.1
Cost Comparison Exhibit

ITEM	VENDOR 1	VENDOR 2	VENDOR 3
Hardware			
Server(s)	None—ASP	$6,802	$4,751
(Separate for PM/EMR if applicable)		Yes	
Software—PM and EMR			
Comments	Subscription	$13,000	$20,000
Modules (extra fees, if applicable)	Limited	Yes	All Included
Monthly ASP Fee	$695		
Onetime activation fee per veterinarian	$1,500		
Comments			
Annual Maintenance			
Software	Included	$2,900	$6,000
Hardware			
Training	$33,500	$30,240	$29,400
On-site			
Comments			
Hours	50	75	80
Data Conversion for PM	$2,000	$2,500	$3,150
Comments			
Hardware Setup and Installation	TBD	TBD	$2,100
Other (detail and price of other features not listed above)			
Comments			
Discounts Negotiated	($7,500)	($8,550)	($12,550)
Total Annualized Price, Year 1	$30,340	$46,892	$52,851
Five-Year Costs			
Year 1	$37,840	$46,892	$52,851
Year 2	$8,340	$2,900	$6,000
Year 3	$8,340	$2,900	$6,000
Year 4	$8,340	$2,900	$6,000
Year 5	$8,340	$2,900	$6,000
Five-Year Total	$71,200	$58,492	$76,851

- Price protection on maintenance fees
- Cost of system
- Addition of future veterinarians/users
- Future recurring fees
- How problems are handled
- How to terminate and exit the relationship

In addition, having a simple problem-resolution clause in the contract will allow the practice and the vendor to work through any difficulties.

As well as these core items, another feature to negotiate is the terms and conditions. The easiest way to negotiate payment terms is to establish a fee schedule that is tied to deployment success. Following is a recommended payment schedule:

- 25 percent due at signing of the contract
- 25 percent due after successful and tested installation of the hardware
- 25 percent due after successful and tested installation of the software
- 25 percent due after successful "go-live"

The contract should also state that maintenance will be paid after the system is implemented. Most vendors try to collect the annual maintenance at the time of signing the contract.

Modify the Contract Language

It should come as no surprise that vendor contracts are not designed with the practice's best interests in mind. This is not to say the vendor is trying to beat customers out of a good deal; it is just that vendors have a lot at risk also, and they can be easy targets for lawsuits. To some extent, it is important for a vendor to be protected from customers who bring unwarranted lawsuits against it, putting it and other customers it supports in jeopardy. It is never, under any circumstances, in a vendor's best interest to have an unsatisfied customer. Most vendors that are serious about staying in business will exhaust all reasonable efforts to keep their customers happy—future sales depend on it.

It is also important to be very respectful and professional during the negotiations. It is never wise to push the vendor to the point of being unreasonable. Remember, the practice will be relying on the vendor for several years. Therefore, mutually acceptable terms and conditions should be the end goal. Following is a list of recommended contract modifications to request from the vendor.

1. **Acceptance period: hardware.** Acceptance will be 90 days after the software is installed on the hardware and all hardware is performing in accordance with expectations. Hardware not properly installed by the vendor will be corrected at the vendor's expense, including travel for on-site work.

2. **Acceptance period: software.** Acceptance will be 90 days after the go-live of each module. Software not properly installed by the vendor (including third-party software) will be corrected at the vendor's expense, including travel for on-site work.

3. **Implementation.** All vendor personnel serving on the implementation team/trainers must have a minimum of one year's employment with the vendor in their current role. The customer does not agree to accept anyone with less than one year of implementation experience. The customer may also request substitute staff, if required.

4. **Support fees.** Support will be charged applicable to what is installed. The support fee does not start until 90 days after go-live. If the practice is installing multiple modules, the vendor will charge support fees for only the portion installed, with a starting point of 90 days after go-live.

5. **Deal-breaker: assignment.** The vendor will allow assignment under the following conditions: a merger, an acquisition, a buyout, a name change, a corporate reorganization, a successor organization, a parent or subsidiary, and another entity within the organization.

6. **Application Service Provider (ASP).** The customer may become an ASP or data center of the software to other veterinarians in the area. The customer will be required to pay the vendor the license fees for the additional users. The vendor may be contracted at its applicable rates to provide training and support services to the practices hosting from the customer.

7. **Future upgrades, new releases, version changes, and mandated modifications.** The vendor will provide continuous/unlimited upgrades/new releases and patches to the customer under the service agreement at no additional cost. Training and installation to support the new releases/upgrades/patches will be covered under the standard maintenance agreement.

8. **Third-party software.** The customer expects the third-party software recommended by the vendor to perform as required and to be compatible with the application. The customer will purchase the recommended software in accordance with the vendor's requirements. The vendor will pay the replacement cost or cost to purchase alternative third-party software if the recommended software does not meet the requirements or if it compromises the performance of the application.

9. **Warranties.** The vendor guarantees to correct any errors, malfunctions, or performance defects in its software within 90 days of the reported problem. If the error cannot be corrected within 90 days or a reasonable substitution cannot be

provided, the customer will be given a 100 percent refund of all expenses paid to the vendor, including hardware and expenses paid for professional services, including travel expenses.

10. **Termination.** The customer may terminate the contract for any reason upon 90 days' notice. Upon termination, the vendor will provide a deconversion file in an ASCII rich text format. The vendor will agree to provide one test tape and one live data tape in the format noted above. At no time may the vendor shut down the software under any circumstances without the customer's prior approval. The customer will be allowed an indefinite amount of time to transition off the software.

11. **Increases in support fees.** The vendor may only increase its support fees at the rate of 1 percent less than the Consumer Price Index (CPI). In addition, the vendor may look back to the prior year only if the CPI is not increased.

12. **Additional support fees.** The cost of unforeseen requests, customization, and other services outside the scope of the agreement will be mutually agreed to.

Now that you have completed a thorough system-selection process, gathered background information to support your negotiations, developed an implementation plan with the vendor, and performed business and legal reviews of the proposed contract, the next step is to discuss with the vendor each issue and the changes you want. This step can be overwhelming, because vendors are very experienced in negotiation. During this step, focus on your priorities, do not get emotional, and remain calm and professional. Purchasing a computer/software system is a major project for any practice, and it is important to ensure that the practice has negotiated a contract to protect its needs and assets.

CONDUCTING A SUCCESSFUL IMPLEMENTATION

Follow a disciplined project management process for working through the implementation plan:

- Create a plan.
- Share the plan.
- Follow the plan.
- Evaluate the plan's effectiveness.
- Revise the plan.

The key to a successful conversion is to create an overall plan for what needs to be accomplished, set a timeline to accomplish these goals, and create a strategy for successful implementation of new technology. Listen to the vendor, successful users, and experts. Work with the vendor's implementation team and empower your project manager to make decisions. Start with the vendor's statement of work (SOW) and progress to a detailed project plan.

There are various ways to implement an electronic health record software solution. Following is a recommended method that will minimize interruptions to the practice and ease veterinarians into going electronic. Make key decisions early. Areas to consider include the following:

- **Import.** Decide which information from the current system should be imported to the new system. This can include demographics, payer files, scheduling, and more. Begin to clean up old files before sending them to be imported.

- **Timing.** Decide on the best time to go live. Most practices prefer to set the date for after a quarter ends and at the start of a new month. If possible (this is highly recommended), try to have veterinarians take vacation and/or reduce the workload at that time. Optimally, close the office for the first day and turn off phones, or see patients in the afternoon only. This will reduce tension and distractions, allowing the staff to focus and get adjusted to the new system. Be sure to tell staff members well in advance not to take vacations or make personal appointments for the week or two before go-live and after. Be realistic with the staff and be clear that a system installation is above their regular duties, requiring longer hours and perhaps working on weekends. Although they may not like to hear this, it is better to establish expectations up front. Encourage them by reassuring them of the benefits of the new system.

- **Training.** Decide who should be trained on what. First, make sure the workflow is correct for the new system. Find out whether the proper personnel are at each job. With a new system, an opportunity opens to evaluate the workflow of the practice. Think of how a patient will be seen and map out what type of staff member should be handling that area. Accomplish this by making a list of employees and their current job functions. Then shuffle them around as needed and list the training they will need. One option is to assign those personnel who are more computer savvy to be the point persons (or trainers) for each area, then train the trainers. It would be helpful for these trainers to have an understanding of how the system is loaded, know from where the data for specific fields are being pulled, and gain an overall view of how everything fits together. That way, if something is not performing properly, problems can usually be solved. Finally, those who are not comfortable with computers should have an opportunity to familiarize themselves with a mouse by playing games or generating e-mails before implementation. In that way they will be better prepared to learn the system and will not need to learn how to navigate a more modern system at the same time.

Software Updates and Continuing Training

The EMR will be updated continually, and new releases will be available that will offer enhancements and fixes to weaknesses (or bugs) in the system. Staff will need continuing education to accompany the software updates and should be given the tools to learn and the time to train to maximize efficiencies. The objective should be to get the most out of the system by using the full capacity of the features offered by the technology. Otherwise, the return on investment will fall short of the goal.

DATA BACKUP AND RECOVERY PROTECTION

Lack of planning for and commitment to data backup and recovery procedures is a widespread issue facing veterinary practices and other small businesses. Data loss is due primarily to hardware failure or disastrous file corruption. The risk associated with data loss can be reduced in several ways. First, if the data are being backed up to a tape drive, an IT professional should perform a test restore from the tapes. Tapes have a shelf life and can go bad after being overwritten many times. Also, store the backup tapes at an off-site location. Although this sounds basic, many businesses back up their data and then store the tape in the same building. If a disaster occurs that damages or destroys the building, such as a fire, flood, or tornado, the tape may be compromised as well. At the very least, use a fireproof safe to store the tape. It is also good to test backup tapes to determine whether they will even help if a server fails. It is easy to record data, but lifting them back up can be a bit trickier.

Although using tapes to back up a system is common, a more modern way of backing up a system is to upload the data to a remote hosting facility or a secondary site. Off-site storage is affordable and, in most cases, data can be restored in a fraction of the time of using a tape, because the secondary system will take over if a failure occurs at the primary site. In addition, many camera-like services are available that take snapshots of data in set intervals for restoration to any point in the day. Finally, consider hosting the practice's server off-site and let the professionals take care of the backups!

Having multiple destinations for data backups can be a lifesaver in the financial management of the veterinary practice.

SUMMARY

Adopting new technology and moving toward a paperless office offers many opportunities for simplifying workflows and enhancing the practice. However, the practice owner is obligated to prepare for the changes in processes and for dealing with vendors. This chapter has provided a basic overview of getting to a good decision and avoiding costly mistakes. By following the advice in this chapter and going through a staged process, the practice will be well on the way to an efficient operational structure for maximizing every aspect of delivering veterinary care.

Glossary

This glossary reviews the key terms associated with financial management, including those specifically related to a veterinary practice. These terms help to standardize and clarify the business of veterinary medicine.

account payable. A *debt* owed to a *creditor*, often as a result of the purchase of merchandise, materials, supplies, or services. An account payable is normally a current *liability*, resulting from day-to-day operations of the practice.

account receivable. A charge against a *debtor*, often from sales or services rendered. This receivable is not necessarily due or past due. An account receivable is the opposite of an *account payable*, and is normally a *current* asset arising from standard business operations.

accounting. A service activity that provides quantitative information, most often financial in nature, about economic entities. The information generated by this activity is intended to be used in economic decision making.

accounting equation. Assets = Liabilities + Owners' Equity OR Assets – Liabilities = Owners' Equity OR Assets – Owners' Equity = Liabilities OR Liabilities + Owners' Equity = Assets.

accounting period. The time period covered by a *financial statement*, including an *income statement* or *statement of cash flows*, usually no less than one month and no more than one year. Financial statements must clearly define the appropriate time periods for which they are relevant.

accounting system. The process, policies, and procedures used for collecting and summarizing financial data in a particular organization.

accounts receivable turnover. The quotient of net *sales* and average *accounts receivable*.

accrual basis of accounting (accrual-based accounting). The method of recognizing *revenue* when goods are delivered or services are provided, regardless of when cash is received. *Expenses* are recognized in the same period the related revenue is recognized.

acquisition cost. The cost of equipment or property plus all expenditures necessary to place and ready that asset for its intended use. Examples of such expenditures are legal fees, transportation charges, and installation costs.

adjusting entry. An entry made to correct an *accounting event* that has been improperly recorded or has not been recorded during the accounting period.

administrative expense. An *expense* related to the business as a whole, such as salaries of the C-suite executives (i.e., the chief executive officer, chief financial officer, chief operating officer, chief technology officer, chief legal officer, etc.), office rental fee, and consulting fees. Administrative expenses can be further broken down into personnel costs, facility costs, and others.

admission of partner. Adding a new business owner (i.e., partner) to the practice. When a new partner joins a *partnership*, the old partnership is legally dissolved and a new one is formed. However, often the old accounting practices are sustained and adjusted only to reflect the newly joined partner. Should a new partner purchase the interest of a different partner, all that is changed is the name on one capital account. If *assets* and *liabilities* are contributed by the new partner, they must be recognized.

aging accounts receivable. A management tool used to classify *accounts receivable* according to the time elapsed since the claim came into being. This is used to determine an entity's uncollectible accounts receivable as of a specific date.

allocate. To divide *revenues* or *expenses* from one account into several accounts, across several periods or among several cost centers.

Americans with Disabilities Act (ADA). The federal law that protects the rights of individuals with disabilities.

amortization. The process of allocating a *debt* to different time periods, as often occurs with a loan, such as a mortgage. The term has also come to mean *writing off* (i.e., liquidating) the cost of an asset. The amortization can be detailed through an *amortization schedule*, which is a table detailing the allocation between *interest* and *principal*.

annuity. Payments of equal amounts, often made at equally spaced intervals.

Application Service Provider (ASP). A third-party entity that manages and distributes software-based services and solutions to customers across a wide area network from a central data center. In essence, ASPs are a way for companies to outsource some or almost all aspects of their information technology needs. They may be commercial ventures that cater to customers, or not-for-profit or government organizations, providing service and support to end users.

appraisal. A valuation of an *asset* or *liability* that involves an expert opinion.

appreciation. An increase in the value of an asset. The opposite of *depreciation*.

arm's-length. A transaction conducted between two parties as though they were independent, even if they are related or otherwise affiliated. An arm's-length transaction ensures an arrangement's compliance with legal guidelines. The basis for a *fair market value* determination.

articles of incorporation. A document filed with a state or other regulatory authority by persons forming a corporation, outlining the management of said corporation. When the document is returned with a certificate of incorporation, it becomes the corporation's charter.

assess. To make an official valuation of an asset.

assets. Everything of value owned by a person, company, or corporation. Assets are generally classified as either *tangible* (including current and fixed assets) or *intangible* (such as goodwill and accounts receivable).

assignment of accounts receivable. Transfer of the legal ownership using *accounts receivable* as collateral. The assignment may be classified as general or specific, depending on the structure of the process.

audit. Systematic inspection of a firm's accounting system and financial records. Also, assessment of a firm's compliance with generally accepted standards set forth by regulatory and governing bodies. *See also* internal audit.

bad debt. Portion of receivables that are *uncollectable*, usually from *accounts receivable* or loans. Bad debt is considered an expense for accounting purposes.

bad debt recovery. Collection of an *account receivable* that was previously written off as *uncollectable*.

balance. The sum of *debit* entries minus the sum of *credit* entries in an account.

balance sheet. A financial statement that lists a firm's assets, liabilities, and owners' equity at a specific point in time.

balloon. A large final payment on a debt. Most *mortgage* and *installment loans* require relatively equal periodic payments. However, some loans (called *balloon loans*) do not fully amortize over the term of the note, thus requiring relatively equal periodic payments but a large final payment due at maturity.

bank balance. The amount in a bank account after various transactions are added and subtracted, as shown on the *bank statement*.

bank reconciliation. The process of comparing the book balance of the cash in a bank account against the bank's statement. Not counting items such as checks issued that have not cleared, deposits that have not cleared, deposits that have not been recorded by the bank, and free of errors made by the bank or the firm, the balance in a firm's accounting records should match the balance of the bank statement.

bank statement. A summary statement sent by the bank to a customer that shows all financial transactions (including deposits, checks cleared, and service charges) for a given period of time, usually one month.

bankrupt. The condition of a company whose *liabilities* exceed the fair market value of its assets. A bankrupt firm is usually insolvent.

bill. An itemized statement of the charges and terms of sale for goods shipped and services rendered. Also a piece of paper currency.

bonus. Premium over normal *wage* or *salary*; usually paid for meritorious performance or increased output.

book. Verb: To recognize a transaction in formal accounting records. Noun, usually plural: The *journals* and *ledgers*. *See also* book value.

book value. The value of an *asset* as carried on the *balance sheet*. Calculated as the cost of an asset less accumulated *depreciation*. Generally used to refer to the *net* amount of an *asset* or group of assets shown in the account.

branch. A division of an organization; often refers to one that is physically separated from the home office of the enterprise, but not organized as a legally separate *subsidiary*.

break-even point. The point at which total *revenues* and total *expenses* are equal, where there is no net loss or gain.

budget. A financial projection used to estimate and control the results of future operations.

burn rate. The amount of *overhead expenses* and other costs in excess of revenue that a firm incurs, usually at the onset of operations. It is ordinarily stated in terms of months.

bylaws. Written rules adopted by the shareholders of a corporation that govern its internal management and specify the procedures for carrying out its functions.

capital. Owners' investment in a business, either in the form of equity investment or long-term debt.

capital asset. Generally, any item that is not bought or sold in standard business operations. This can include land, building, furniture, and equipment.

capital budget. A plan of proposed outlays for acquiring long-term *assets* and the means by which these assets will be financed.

capital gain. The profit that results when the selling price of a *capital asset* exceeds the purchase price. If the *capital asset* has been held for a sufficiently long period of time before sale, then the tax on the gain is computed at a rate lower than is used for other gains and ordinary income.

capital lease. A lease used to finance an *asset* for the majority of its useful life. Both the *liability* and the *asset* are recognized on the lessee's *balance sheet*. Also called a finance lease.

capital loss. A loss incurred when the selling price of a *capital asset* is lower than the purchase price. Opposite of *capital gain*.

capitalization of earnings. The process of valuing a business by computing the net present value of its predicted future *net income*.

cash. Money in the form of currency, such as coins or paper bills, that is typically kept on hand. A common form of cash kept on hand is referred to as *petty cash*.

cash basis of accounting (cash-based accounting). A system of accounting in which *revenues* are recorded when cash is received and *expenses* are recognized as payments are made. No attempt is made to match *revenues* and *expenses* in determining *income* in a fixed *accounting period*.

cash budget. Estimation of cash *receipts* and *disbursements* for a business for a specific period of time. This budget is used to determine whether a firm has enough money to maintain standard operations and whether money is being used in unproductive capacities.

cash flow. Change in a cash account over a period of time, usually as the result of financing, operating, or investing. Measuring cash flow can be used for future planning and assessment of the financial health of an organization.

cash receipts journal. A specialized *journal* used to record all *receipts* of cash.

certified check. A type of check issued by a bank that guarantees there are sufficient reserves to fund the amount noted on the check. After it is issued, the check becomes an obligation of the bank.

chart of accounts. A systematic list of all accounts in a general ledger, each accompanied by a reference number.

check. "A *draft* or order upon a bank or banking house purporting to be drawn upon a deposit of funds for the payment at all events of a certain sum of money to a certain person therein named or to him or his order or to bearer and payable instantly on demand" (Federal Reserve Board definition). A check must contain the phrase "pay to the order of." The amount shown on the check's face must be clearly readable, and it must have the signature of the drawer. Checks need not be dated, although they usually are. The *balance* in the *cash account* is usually reduced when a check is issued, not later when it clears the bank and actually reduces the money in the bank.

check register. A *journal* to record *checks* that are issued.

close. To transfer the balance of a *temporary* or *contra* or *adjunct* account to the main account to which it relates (e.g., to transfer *revenue* and *expense* accounts directly, or through the *income summary*, to an *owners' equity* account, or to transfer *purchase discounts* to purchases). To *close* the books entails the above, usually done only once each year, at the end of the fiscal year.

closing entries. At the end of the accounting period, the *entries* that accomplish the transfer of balances in *temporary accounts* to the related *income summary account* and *retained earnings account*.

coinsurance. Insurance that protects against hazards, such as fire or water damage. In property insurance, coinsurance can take the form of a penalty by the insurance carrier wherein the insured may not collect the full amount of insurance for a loss unless the insurance policy covers at least some specified coinsurance percentage, usually about 80 percent of the *replacement cost* of the property. Coinsurance clauses induce the owner to carry full, or nearly full, coverage.

COLA. Cost of Living Adjustment. *See also* indexation.

collateral. Security or guarantee (often an *asset*) pledged by a *borrower* that will be given up if the *loan* is not repaid.

collectable. Capable of being converted into *cash* now or at a later date.

commercial paper. An unsecured, short-term note issued by corporate borrowers with a fixed maturity of 1 to 270 days. Corporations often use these notes for meeting *short-term liabilities* and financing *accounts receivable*.

commission. Remuneration to employees based on an activity rate, such as services rendered or products sold; usually expressed as a percentage.

comparative (financial) statements. *Financial statements* in a consistent format showing information for the same company for various periods of time, usually two successive years. Nearly all published financial statements are in this form. Contrast with *historical summary*.

compound interest. Accumulated interest calculated on *principal* plus previously undistributed interest.

consolidated financial statements. Statements issued by legally separate companies that share common ownership. These statements show an aggregated financial position and income as they would appear if the companies were one economic *entity*.

Consumer Price Index (CPI). An index of prices used to measure the change in the cost of basic goods and services in comparison with a fixed base period. Also called cost-of-living index.

contributed capital. Amount paid to a company in exchange for an ownership interest. Also called *paid-in capital*.

contribution margin. *Revenue* less *variable expenses*. Gross operating margin per unit sold.

control system. A device or set of devices for ensuring that actions are carried out according to plan or for safeguarding *assets*.

controller. A person who manages accounting, financial reporting, and internal controls in an organization. This title is often given to the chief accountant of an organization. Also known as *comptroller*.

corporation. A business organization authorized by a state (in a process called incorporation) to operate under the rules of the entity's *charter*.

correcting entry. An *adjusting entry* whereby an improperly recorded *transaction* is properly recorded. The entry always involves an *income statement* account (revenue or expense) as well as a *balance sheet* account (asset or liability).

cost. The value, measured by the *price* paid or required to be paid, needed to acquire *goods* or *services*.

cost center. Part of an organization that does not directly increase profits but adds to the expense of running that organization.

cost of goods sold (COGS). A figure on the income statement that reflects the cost of products sold to consumers in the primary business activity of an organization.

credit. Noun: An entry on the right-hand side of an account ledger. Verb: To make an entry on the right-hand side of an account ledger. It records increases in *liabilities, owners'* equity, revenues, and *gains* and records decreases in *assets* and *expenses*. Also the ability or right to buy or borrow in return for a promise to pay later.

credit memorandum. A commercial document used by a seller to inform a buyer that the buyer's *account receivable* is being credited (reduced) because of *damages, errors, returns,* or *allowances*. Also, the form provided to a depositor by a bank to indicate that the depositor's balance is being increased because of some event other than a deposit.

current asset. A *balance sheet* item equaling cash and other *assets* that are expected to be converted into cash, usually within one year. Current *assets* include *cash, cash equivalents, marketable securities, accounts receivable, inventory,* and *prepaid expenses*.

current funds. *Cash* and other *liquid assets* readily convertible into cash.

current liability. An organization's debts or other obligations that must be discharged within a short time, usually the *earnings cycle* or one year. *Current liabilities* appear on the *balance sheet*.

current replacement cost. The price paid to replace an existing asset with an identical asset (in the same condition and with the same service potential).

customers' ledger. The *ledger* that shows accounts receivable of individual customers. It is the *subsidiary ledger* for the *controlling account*, accounts receivable.

debit. Noun: An entry on the left-hand side of an account ledger. Verb: To make an entry on the left-hand side of an account ledger. It records increases in *assets* and decreases in *liabilities* and *net worth*. A debit is the opposite of a credit.

debit memorandum. A document used by a seller to inform a buyer that the seller is debiting (increasing) the amount of the buyer's *account receivable*. Also, the document provided by a bank to a depositor to indicate that the depositor's *balance* is being decreased because of some event other than payment for a *check*, such as monthly service charges or the printing of checks. Also called a *debit note*.

debt. An amount owed. The general name for *loans, notes, bonds,* and *mortgages* that are evidence of amounts owed and have definite payment dates.

deferral. An accrual accounting process wherein past *cash receipts* and *payments* are not recognized on the *income statement* until some later period. Deferred revenues are recognized as *liabilities* and deferred expenses are recognized as *assets*.

defined contribution plan. A *pension or retirement plan,* such as a 401(k) or 403(b) plan, to which an employer makes cash contributions (either a set amount or a percentage) to eligible individual employee *accounts* under the terms of a formalized plan.

depreciation. The process of allocating the cost of an asset across the time period for which it provides benefit (known as the asset's *depreciable* or *useful life*). Depreciation is a non-cash expense.

disbursement. Payment of a debt or expense by *cash* or by *check*.

double entry. System of financial accounting wherein each transaction is recorded in at least two accounts to maintain the equality of the accounting equation; each entry results in recording equal amounts of *debits* and *credits*.

EBITDA (earnings before interest, taxes, depreciation, and amortization)). An approximate measure of a company's operating cash flow based on data from its income statement, frequently used in accounting ratios for comparison with other companies.

equity. A claim to *assets*. Ownership interest in a corporation that takes the form of common or preferred stock.

ERISA. Employment Retirement Income Security Act of 1974. The federal statute that sets minimum standards and other requirements for *pension plans,* as well as the rules on federal income tax effects related to these pension plans.

expense. Outflow of cash or other *assets* in producing *revenue* or carrying out other activities that are part of an entity's *operations*. Expenses result in a decrease in *owners' equity*.

fair market value. Value (price) negotiated at *arm's length* between a willing buyer and a willing seller, each acting rationally in his or her own self-interest with knowledge of all relevant facts.

FICA. Federal Insurance Contributions Act. Social Security and Medicare payroll taxes and benefits are collected under this act.

financial projection. Planning process that creates estimates of *sales* and *revenue, expenses, cost of goods sold,* and short- and long-term *debt.* This process aids in budgeting and outlining future financing needs.

financial statements. Documentation of an organization's financial activities. These statements include the *balance sheet, income statement, statement of retained earnings,* and *statement of cash flow,* as well as any notes thereto.

fiscal year. A period of 12 consecutive months chosen by a business as the *accounting period* for annual reports. May or may not be aligned with the calendar year.

fixed cost (expense). An *expenditure* or *expense* that does not vary with production, sales, or volume of activity. Fixed costs include rent, insurance, property tax, and interest expense.

float. *Checks* whose amounts have been *added* to a depositor's bank account, but not yet subtracted from the *drawer's* bank account. *Free float* refers to the number of shares of a publicly owned company available for trading.

foreclosure. The legal proceedings that can occur when a borrower fails to make a required payment on a *mortgage.* During these proceedings, the lender obtains a court-ordered termination of the borrower's equitable right of redemption and takes possession of the property for its use or sale.

full-time-equivalent (FTE). Ratio of total number of paid hours during a period (e.g., part-time, full-time, contracted) divided by the number of working hours in that period, Mondays through Fridays.

fully vested. The condition of a *pension plan* when an employee (or his or her estate) has rights to all the benefits purchased with the employer's contributions to the plan, even if the employee is not employed by this employer at the time of death or retirement.

FUTA. Federal Unemployment Tax Act. Payroll or employment tax paid only by an employer. Although the tax is not deducted from the employee's wage, the amount paid by the employer is based on each employee's wages.

Generally Accepted Accounting Principles (GAAP). Authoritative rules, practices, and conventions meant to provide both broad guidelines and detailed procedures for preparing financial statements and handling specific accounting situations. They provide objective standards for judging and comparing financial data and their presentation, and limit the directors' freedom in showing an unrealistic picture through creative accounting. An auditor must certify that the provisions of GAAP have been followed in reporting an organization's financial data in order for them to be accepted by investors, lenders, and tax authorities.

general journal. The formal record wherein *double entry* bookkeeping entries are recognized through matching *debits* and *credits* (thus ensuring the maintenance of the *accounting equation*).

general ledger. The formal *accounting record* containing all of an organization's financial statement accounts. Also called the *nominal ledger*.

goodwill. An *intangible asset* listed on an organization's *balance sheet*. It represents the value of an organization's reputable brand name, positive customer relations, patents, and other nonphysical assets. Goodwill can reflect the amount paid for an organization beyond its *book value* during an acquisition.

grandfather clause. An exemption in new accounting pronouncements that exempts transactions that occurred before a given date from the new accounting requirements.

gross. An amount of money not adjusted or reduced by deductions or subtractions. Contrast with *net*.

gross margin. Total sales less the *cost of goods sold*. Also called *gross profit*.

holding company. A company that confines its activities to owning other companies' outstanding *stock*. A holding company can supervise and manage other companies through ownership of a controlling interest in the companies whose stock it holds.

in the black. Operating at a profit.

in the red. Operating at a loss.

income. "Increases in economic benefits during the accounting period in the form of inflows or enhancements of assets or decreases in liabilities that result in increases in equity, other than those relating to contributions from equity participants" (International Accounting Standards Board definition). *Income* is synonymous with *revenue*, but is often used as a shorthand reference for *net income*.

income accounts. *Revenue* and *expense accounts*.

income statement. The summary statement of *revenues* and *expenses* for a period of time, ending with *net income*. Also called the *profit and loss statement (P&L)*.

income tax. An annual tax levied by the federal and other governments on the income of people, corporations, and other legal entities.

indexation. Technique used to mitigate the effects of *inflation*. Income payments fixed in law or contracts are adjusted using a *price index* when they change as a given measure of price changes. This serves to transfer risk from the payee to the payer.

inflation. Increase in the general price of products and services over a period of time.

information system. A system, either formal or informal, for collecting, processing, storing, and communicating data. The people, records, and processes that comprise this system can be used to drive managerial decision making.

Information Technology (IT). The development, installation, and implementation of computer systems and applications.

installment. Portion of a *debt* paid in successive payments at predetermined intervals.

insurance. A risk-reward relationship that reimburses for specific covered losses in exchange for the payment of premiums.

intangible asset. A nonphysical asset that provides an organization an exclusive or preferred position in the marketplace. Examples of intangible assets are copyrights, patents, trademarks, goodwill, organization costs, business methodologies, brand recognition, intellectual property, computer programs, government licenses, leases, franchises, mailing lists, exploration permits, import and export permits, construction permits, and marketing quotas.

interest. The charge or cost for using borrowed assets. The interest rate (generally expressed as a percentage) is the fee paid per period, usually one year, for the use of the borrowed funds.

internal audit. An analysis conducted by employees to evaluate an organization's compliance with business processes and procedures and to determine whether or not *internal controls* are effective. An external audit is conducted by a CPA.

Internal Rate of Return (IRR). The rate of discount on an investment that equates the present value of the investment's cash outflows with the present value of the investment's cash inflows. Internal rate of return is analogous to yield to maturity for a bond.

inventory. Noun: The raw materials, supplies, work in process, and completely finished goods that serve as part of an organization's total *assets*. Verb: To calculate the *cost of goods* on hand at a given time or to create a detailed list of all items on hand.

investment. An expenditure to acquire property or other assets in order to produce *revenue*; a redirection of current resources made in anticipation of creating future benefits.

IRS. Internal Revenue Service. Agency of the United States Department of the Treasury responsible for collecting income and certain other taxes and administering the Internal Revenue Code enacted by Congress.

journal. The document in which business transactions are originally recorded as they occur. The book of entry prior to transfer to the *ledger*.

journal entry. The initial recording of a business transaction in an organization's accounting system. Entries are made in a *journal* and list equal *debits* and *credits*, with an explanation of the transaction, if necessary.

key performance indicators (KPIs). Key business statistics, such as number of new orders, cash collection efficiency, and return on investment (ROI), that measure a company's performance in critical areas. KPIs show the progress (or lack of it) toward realizing the company's objectives or strategic plans by monitoring activities that (if not properly performed) would likely cause severe losses or outright failure.

kiting. The wrongful and illegal practice of taking advantage of the *float*, the time that elapses between the deposit of a *check* in one financial institution and its collection at another, for the purpose of increasing financial leverage.

lapping scheme. A fraudulent accounting method wherein the *accounts receivable* section of an organization's *balance sheet* is altered to mask theft. For example, an employee could steal cash sent in by a customer. The theft from the first customer is concealed by using cash received from a second customer. The theft from the second customer is concealed by using the cash received from a third customer, and so on. The process could be continued until the thief returns the funds or makes the theft permanent by creating a fictitious *expense* or receivable write-off, or until the fraud is discovered.

lease. A legal document or oral arrangement calling for the lessee (user) to pay the lessor (owner) for the possession and use of an *asset*.

leasehold improvement. An *improvement* to a leased asset often resulting in an increase in that asset's value. Should be *depreciated* over the life of the lease or the improvement.

ledger. The principal book for recording accounts and business transactions.

liability. An obligation that requires an individual or company to pay a definite (or reasonably definite) amount at a definite (or reasonably definite) time in order to settle a debt. Liabilities are recorded on an organization's *balance sheet* and include accounts payable, notes payable, accrued expenses, deferred revenues, unearned revenue, and payable for wages, taxes, and interest.

limited partner. A member of a *partnership* who does not take part in the management of the organization and has limited personal *liability* for the debts of the partnership; every partnership must have at least one *general partner* who is fully liable. The limited partner is also called the nominal partner.

liquid assets. *Cash, current marketable securities,* and sometimes *current receivables*; assets that can be converted into cash quickly and easily.

loan. A debt instrument wherein the owner of an asset (lender) allows another party (borrower) use of the asset for a period of time under an agreement that the borrower will return the asset and often make payments for the use of the asset. Generally the asset being lent is *cash* and the payment for its use is *interest*.

loss. A condition wherein *expenses* exceed *revenues*. Negative *income* for a period or single transaction. An expenditure that produced no *revenue*.

margin. *Revenue* less specified *expenses*. Also known as *profit margin*.

merger. The combining of two or more businesses into a single economic entity.

Modified Accelerated Cost Recovery System (MACRS). The depreciation method used since 1986 for deducting the value of depreciable property other than real estate. MACRS depreciation is faster than straight-line depreciation. MACRS depreciation is less favorable than the prior ACRS system.

money market account (MMA). Special savings account that pays a fluctuating interest rate that, on average, is higher than the interest rate on ordinary savings accounts. However, a certain minimum credit balance must be maintained in an MMA, and only a limited number of checks can be written on it in a month, though usually there is no limit on transfer of funds over the bank's counter or through automated teller machines (ATMs). An MMA balance, like an ordinary savings account balance, is covered under deposit insurance.

mortgage. A legal contract between a borrower and a lender wherein the lender provides a loan that is secured by the borrower's real estate.

negotiable. Legally capable of being sold or transferred by endorsement and delivery. Typically used in reference to *checks* and *notes*.

net. The amount remaining after all relevant deductions.

net income. Gross profit less operating expenses, costs, and taxes. Also referred to as *the bottom line*.

net loss. A condition in which *expenses* and *losses* incurred in a given period exceed the *revenues* and *gains* of that same period.

net present value (NPV). Difference between the present value (PV) of the future cash flows from an investment and the amount of investment. Present value of the expected cash flows is computed by discounting them at the required rate of return (also called minimum rate of return). For example, an investment of $1,000 today at 10 percent will yield $1,100 at the end of the year; therefore, the present value of $1,100 at the desired rate of return (10 percent) is $1,000. The amount of investment ($1,000 in this example) is deducted from this figure to arrive at NPV, which here is zero ($1,000 to $1,000). A zero NPV means the project repays original investment plus the required rate of return. A positive NPV means a better return, and a negative NPV means a worse return, than the return from zero NPV. It is one of the two discounted cash flow (DCF) techniques (the other is internal rate of return) used in comparative appraisal of investment proposals where the flow of income varies over time.

nonprofit corporation. An incorporated *entity*, such as a hospital, with shareholders who do not share in the earnings. This type of organization usually emphasizes providing programs and services (often for public benefit) rather than maximizing income.

note. An unconditional written promise by the payee (borrower) to pay a specific sum on demand or at a certain future time. Also called a *promissory note*.

OASDHI. Old Age, Survivors, Disability, and Health Insurance. A federal program created by the Social Security Act of 1935 to provide benefits to qualified retirees, their spouses and dependents, and some disabled workers.

operating. An adjective used to refer to *revenue* and *expense items* relating to an organization's principal line of business.

OSHA. Occupational Safety and Health Administration. An agency of the United States Department of Labor created by Congress under the Occupational Safety and Health Act. This agency issues and enforces standards for safe and healthy working conditions in commerce and industry.

out-of-pocket. An adjective that refers to an e*xpenditure* or *outlay* (usually in cash) that may or may not be reimbursed at a later time.

outstanding. Amount left unpaid or uncollected. Value owed as a *debt*.

overdraft. A withdrawal in excess of the available balance. Often refers to a check written on a checking account that contains insufficient funds to cover the amount of the check.

overhead costs. Expenditures and expenses associated with the ongoing operations of a business. These costs are necessary to maintain the existence of a business and are not directly associated with the production or sale of goods and services.

P&L. Profit and loss statement. The summary statement of *revenues* and *expenses* for a period of time, ending with *net income*. Another term for *income statement*.

partnership. Relationship between two or more people who share resources and operations in a jointly run organization. Partners (also called owners) share the profits and losses incurred by the business in which they have invested.

payable. A *liability* that a company owes for goods or services purchased on *credit*.

payroll taxes. A portion of the employee's wages or salary withheld by the employer for the purpose of paying local, state, and federal taxing authorities to fund programs such as Social Security, Medicare, and unemployment compensation.

pension fund. A fund containing assets that are to be paid to retired, ex-employees as an *annuity*, typically held by an independent trustee and not to be considered an *asset* of the employer.

pension plan. Details or provisions of an employment contract for setting aside *annuities* or other benefits to be accessed by employees after they retire to sustain their standard of living.

petty cash fund. A small fund of cash maintained for incidental expenditures (e.g., office supplies).

practice management system (PMS). A category of software that deals with the day-to-day practice operations. Such software frequently allows users to capture patient demographics, schedule appointments, perform billing tasks, maintain inventory control, complete payroll, conduct accounting functions, maintain clinical record keeping, and generate reports.

prime rate. The *interest rate* charged by banks for loans to their stable and creditworthy customers.

principal. The original amount of a *debt* on which *interest* is calculated. Also commonly used to describe the person who hires the agent when the owner is absent in a *principal-agent* relationship.

prior-period adjustment. A *debit* or *credit* made directly to *retained earnings* prior to the start of the current period so that it has no direct impact on income for the current period.

pro forma statements. Hypothetical statements. Financial statements as they would appear if some event, such as a *merger* or increased production and sales, were to occur.

profit center. A business unit or set of activities that generates *revenue*; contrast with *cost center.*

profit-sharing plan. An *incentive plan,* which can take various forms, wherein the employer contributes an amount for the benefit of the employee based on the *net income* of the company.

promissory note. A written agreement in which a party agrees to pay a predetermined sum of money on demand or at a specified future date. *See also* note.

prorate. To *allocate* or assess in proportion to a baseline.

purchase order. A document used to request that a *vendor* provide a good or a service in return for payment.

ratio. The result of dividing one number by another. Ratios are generally used to assess aspects of profitability, solvency, and liquidity of a business entity. The three most commonly used financial ratios are to summarize some aspect of *operations* for a period, to summarize some aspect of *financial position* at a given point in time, and to relate some aspect of operations to a financial position.

receipt. The act of receiving *cash.*

rent. A charge or payment, usually in a fixed amount and for a set period of time, for the occupancy or use of land or buildings belonging to another person or corporation.

retained earnings. Revenue that is kept by a company for reinvestment in the company or to pay off debt. This money is not paid out to shareholders as *dividends.*

revenue. The amount of money generated by the company from the sale of goods or property (*tangible* or *intangible*) or from services provided.

risk. A measure of uncertainty and its impact on *return on investment.* Most people prefer less risk to more risk; therefore in financial markets, investments with increased levels of risk are expected to return a higher yield or rate of return than investments with lower levels of risk.

risk premium. Extra compensation paid to an employee or additional *interest* paid to a lender, above the normal amounts, in return for their engaging in activities with greater than normal risk.

ROI. Return on investment. A measure of profitability used to refer to a single project and expressed as a ratio; *revenue* generated divided by the average *cost* of *assets* consumed as part of the project.

salary. Fixed compensation for services that is earned and paid on a regular basis but not based on an hourly rate. Contrast with *wage.*

sale. A transaction wherein *goods, services,* or *property* (tangible or intangible) is delivered to a customer in return for cash or an obligation to pay; *revenue.*

simple interest. *Interest* calculated only on *principal,* not compounded or added to the principal or paid to the lender. Interest = Principal × Interest Rate × Time. Contrast with *compound interest.*

SOAP. An acronym for Subjective, Objective, Assessment Plan identifying the most common data entry format used by veterinary practices. These data are generally maintained in the progress notes portion of a medical record.

Social Security taxes. Taxes levied by the federal government on employers and employees to provide funds to pay retired persons, or their beneficiaries, who are entitled to receive such payments, either because they paid Social Security taxes themselves or are determined to be eligible by the federal government.

sole proprietorship. A business structure in which *owners' equity* belongs to a single person.

spreadsheet. A *worksheet* organized with columns and rows to enable two-way classification of financial data.

Statement of Work (SOW). Detailed description of the specific services or tasks a contractor is required to perform under a contract. SOW is usually incorporated in a contract, indirectly by reference or directly as an attachment.

SWOT. An acronym for Strengths, Weaknesses, Opportunities, and Threat, designating an analytical tool for auditing an organization and its environment. It is the first stage of planning and helps strategists to focus on key issues. Strengths and weaknesses are internal factors. Opportunities and threats are external factors.

T-account. Account formed by two perpendicular lines forming the letter "T" with the title above the horizontal line. *Debits* are captured to the left of the center line, and *credits* to the right.

take-home pay. The amount of *wages* or *salary* minus the deductions for *income taxes, Social Security taxes,* contributions to benefits plans, and dues.

tax credit. A reduction in *liability* that is otherwise payable.

tax deduction. A reduction from *revenues* and *gains* to determine taxable income. Tax deductions are technically different from tax *exemptions,* but both are used to reduce *gross income* in determining taxable income.

taxable income. *Income* subject to taxation that is computed according to applicable local, state, or federal laws or regulations. *Pretax income* refers to income before taxes on the income statement in financial reports.

tickler file. A collection of *vouchers* or other time-sensitive documents arranged chronologically in order to remind the person in charge of certain duties to make payments (or to do other tasks) in order of occurrence.

trial balance. A listing of all accounts with *debit* and *credit* balances in *double-entry* bookkeeping, which when totaled separately are equal.

underwriter. An intermediary between the issuer of a security and the purchasing public. The intermediary agrees to purchase an entire *security issue* for a specified price to resell to others.

value. Monetary worth; an amount of goods, services, or money considered to be a reasonable equivalent for something else. *See also* fair market value.

variance. The discrepancy between actual and budgeted or planned costs, expenditures, or expenses.

vendor. A party that provides a good or a service in return for money.

vested. The condition of an employee's *pension plan* benefits that are not contingent on the employee's continued employment by the employer because the employee has worked a minimum period for vesting set by the employer.

veterinary time equivalent (VTE). A method of assigning labor expenses on the basis of veterinary staffing expense. This allows a practice to calculate labor expenses for procedures using veterinary expense as a standard.

wage. Compensation based on time worked or output of product by manual labor. *See also* take-home pay.

warranty. An obligation or guarantee that is stated or legally implied by the seller and that often provides for a specific remedy such as repair or replacement in the event the article or service fails to meet a given standard.

weighted average. An average computed by applying a weight to each value so that it is not treated as equal to other values.

withholding. A portion of an employee's *salary* or *wages*, usually for local, state, or federal *income taxes*, to be remitted by the employer, in the employee's name, to the taxing authority.

write down. Downward revision of the value of an asset to reflect its market value, which has dropped below the *book value*. The amount by which the *book value* is reduced is charged against the earnings as an expense or loss.

write off. To *charge* an asset to *expense* or *loss* in order to reduce the value of one's assets and earnings.

Index

About the Authors

Justin Chamblee, CPA, MAcc, is a manager in Financial Services for Coker Group. Chamblee works with clients in a variety of financial areas and ventures, including valuations, appraisals, mergers and acquisitions, pro formas, expert witness testimony, and financial assessments. His strong background in accounting, financial analysis, and problem solving gives him insight into clients' unique financial needs and goals.

Prior to joining Coker, Chamblee was a senior associate at PricewaterhouseCoopers, where he worked on financial statement audits for multi-billion-dollar publicly traded companies, including the review of documents to be filed with the Securities and Exchange Commission. He worked closely with executives, such as the controller and director of financial reporting; was as an audit team member solving complex accounting issues; performed technical research; and served on the coaching staff.

Chamblee has contributed to Coker publications, including *Physician Entrepreneurs: Strength in Numbers—Consolidation and Collaboration Strategies to Grow Your Practice* (HealthLeaders Media, 2008) and *Physician Entrepreneurs: Going Retail—Business Strategies to Grow Beyond Traditional Practice Models* (HealthLeaders Media, 2007).

Chamblee holds a bachelors of business administration (BBA) in accounting and a master of accounting (MAcc) from Abilene Christian University. He is licensed as a CPA in Texas and is a member of the American Institute of Certified Public Accountants.

Max Reiboldt, CPA, provides sound financial and strategic solutions to hospitals, medical practices, health systems, and other health-care entities through keen analysis and problem solving. Working with organizations of all sizes, Reiboldt engages in consulting projects with organizations nationwide. His expertise encompasses employee and physician employment and compensation, physician/hospital affiliation initiatives, business and strategic planning, mergers and acquisitions, practice operational assessments, ancillary services development, PHO/IPA/MSO development, practice appraisals, and negotiations for acquisitions and sales. He also performs financial analyses for health-care entities as well as buy/sell agreements and planning arrangements for medical practices.

He is president and CEO of Coker Group and has led the firm's growth since the late 1990s to its position today as one of the leading health-care consulting firms in the

United States and abroad. He is a prolific author and accomplished public speaker on health-care management topics.

Reiboldt has authored many of Coker Group's more than fifty books. Recent titles include *Physician Entrepreneurs: Strength in Numbers—Consolidation and Collaboration Strategies to Grow Your Practice* (HealthLeaders Media, 2008) and *Physician Entrepreneurs: Going Retail—Business Strategies to Grow Beyond Traditional Practice Models* (HealthLeaders Media, 2007).

A graduate of Harding University, Reiboldt is a licensed CPA in Georgia and Louisiana and a member of the American Institute of Certified Public Accountants, Healthcare Financial Management Association, and American Society of Appraisers.